Competences for Pharmacy Education and Practice in Europe

Competences for Pharmacy Education and Practice in Europe

Selected Articles Published by MDPI

MDPI • Basel • Beijing • Wuhan • Barcelona • Belgrade

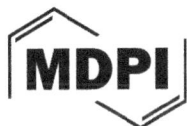

MDPI

Editorial Office
MDPI
St. Alban-Anlage 66
Basel, Switzerland

This is a reprint of articles published online by the open access publisher MDPI from 2013 to 2016 (available at: http://www.mdpi.com).

For citation purposes, cite each article independently as indicated on the article page online and as indicated below:

LastName, A.A.; LastName, B.B.; LastName, C.C. Article Title. *Journal Name* **Year**, *Article Number*, Page Range.

ISBN 978-3-03897-093-4 (Pbk)
ISBN 978-3-03897-094-1 (PDF)

Contents

Preface to "Competences for Pharmacy Education and Practice in Europe"

One of the main aspirations of the European Union (EU) is the development of a pan-European health system in all member states, with unhindered access to quality care. The PHAR-QA "Quality Assurance in European Pharmacy Education and Training" project explored the realities surrounding this idea in the area of pharmacy. This book assembles a series of papers, already published in the journal "Pharmacy", that describe the project: its origins, design, implementation, results, interpretation, and perspectives.

Prelude

The papers assembled in the prelude describe the existing problems and, hence, the need for the PHAR-QA project.

A first paper looked at the heterogeneity in pharmacy education in the EU. EU directives assume that the harmonisation of pharmacy education across the EU provides the basis for the mutual recognition of diplomas—and, beyond that, for the harmonisation of quality healthcare in the EU. However, a study by the European Association of Faculties of Pharmacy (EAFP) in 1994 showed that there was a large variability in the course content. In 2011, a precursor of PHAR-QA, the PHARMINE "Pharmacy Education in Europe" project, investigated whether the variability had decreased, using a methodology similar to that used by the EAFP in 1994. Information from across all EU countries on the number of contact hours in specific subject areas in 1994 and 2011 was compared. The results showed that there had been no increase in the harmonisation of the course content over the 17 year period.

A second paper looked at what already existed in terms of quality assurance and competence training in pharmacy education and training in several EU states. The PHAR-QA consortium analysed quality assurance (and degree accreditation systems) in 10 EU countries and looked at how far such systems have evolved from a "resources and curriculum" basis towards a "competences" basis. It was found that quality assurance was based primarily on resources and management, not on competences. Furthermore, the systems were national, not pan-European. Rather than checking whether pharmacists throughout the EU have the same competences to fulfil their present and future tasks, the quality assurance systems and the accompanying measures for degree accreditation evaluated curriculum structure (number of contact hours in specific subject areas, etc.) and resources (length of the course, etc.).

On this basis, PHAR-QA set out to produce a European series of competences for pharmacy education and training that could be used for the harmonisation of the pharmacy degree courses and pharmacy practice.

Design, implementation, and results of the two rounds of the PHAR-QA study

The third, "methodological" paper was descriptive, outlining how PHAR-QA would define competences and establish a quality assurance system based on them. This paper also considered the various stakeholders, such as staff and students of EU departments. It was considered that the final stake holder is the European patient who would benefit from better pharmaceutical services with better medications and pharmaceutical care.

The fourth paper set out the goals of the PHAR-QA project for the production of a European framework for a quality assurance system based on competences for pharmacy practice. The PHAR-QA framework is intended to be European, consultative, and encompassing the various aspects of pharmacy practice. In the first PHAR-QA round, using the proposals for competences produced by our previous PHARMINE project together with those of other sources, three university professors of pharmacy (Authors 2 through 4) produced a list of three major competency domains that reflect the activities of the practitioners: Patient Care Competences, Personal Competences and Management, and Organizational Structure Competences. Each domain was subdivided into nine, nine, and eight competencies, respectively, for a total of 27 major competencies that were further subdivided into an average of five supporting competences per major competence, giving a total of 140 proposals for competences for pharmacy practice. The 27 major competences and 140 proposals were ranked by an expert panel of seven university professors of pharmacy (Authors 5 through 11). The panel also commented on the proposed competences. On the basis of the ranks and comments, a list of 68 proposals for competences was produced. This list was then examined by the expert panel, and a new version based on their comments was produced. The latter process was repeated twice, using the Delphi methodology. The 68 proposals were ranked by the pharmacy community.

The fifth paper described the results of the first PHAR-QA round of the ranking of competences required for practice performed by EU academia, students, and practicing pharmacists. The results showed that competences in the areas of "drug interactions", "need for drug treatment", and "provision of information and service" were ranked the highest, whereas those in the areas of "ability to design and conduct research" and "development and production of medicines" were ranked lower. For the latter two categories, industrial pharmacists ranked them higher than the other five groups.

The sixth paper presented the results of the second European Delphi round of the ranking of competences for pharmacy practice and compared these data to those of the first round, already published (see fifth paper above). A comparison of the numbers of respondents, distribution by age group, country of residence, etc., showed that, whilst the student population of respondents changed from round 1 to 2, the populations of the professional groups (community, hospital and industrial pharmacists, pharmacists in other occupations, and academics) were more stable. Results were given for the consensus of ranking and the scores of ranking of 50 competences for pharmacy practice. This two-stage, large-scale Delphi process harmonized and validated the PHAR-QA framework and provided a sound base for the adoption by the pharmacy profession of a framework proposed by the academic pharmacy community. The process of evaluation and validation of the ranking of competences by the pharmacy profession is now complete, and the PHAR-QA consortium put forward a definitive PHAR-QA framework of competences for pharmacy practice.

Interpretation of the PHAR-QA results

A seventh paper looked at a subsection of the PHAR-QA first round data viz the opinions of 241 European academics (who provide pharmacy education) and of 258 European community pharmacists (who apply it) on 68 competences for pharmacy practice. Academics and community pharmacy practitioners recognized the importance of the notion of patient care competences, underlining the nature of the pharmacist as a specialist of medicines. The survey revealed certain discrepancies. Academics placed substantial emphasis on research, pharmaceutical technology, regulatory aspects of quality, etc., but these were ranked much lower by community pharmacists, who concentrated more on patient care competences. In a sub-analysis of the data, it was evaluated how perceptions may have changed since the 1980s, and the notions of competence and pharmaceutical care were introduced. This was done by splitting both groups into respondents <40 and >40 years of age. The results for the subgroups were essentially statistically the same but with some different qualitative tendencies. The results were discussed in the light of the different conceptions of the professional identity of the pharmacist.

An eighth paper studied the hospital pharmacy subsection in the PHAR-QA first round data, looking at the way in which hospital pharmacists rank the fundamental competences for pharmacy practice. European hospital pharmacists (n = 152) ranked 68 competences for pharmacy practice of two types (personal and patient care), arranged into 13 clusters. The results were compared to those obtained from community pharmacists (n = 258). Generally, hospital and community pharmacists ranked competences in a similar way. Nevertheless, differences were detected. The higher focus of hospital pharmacists on knowledge of the different areas of science as well as on laboratory tests reflected the idea of a hospital pharmacy specialization. The difference was also visible in the field of drug production. This is a necessary competence in hospitals with requests for drugs for rare diseases, as well as pediatric and oncologic drugs. Hospital pharmacists gave entrepreneurship a lower score and cost-effectiveness a higher one than community pharmacists. This reflects the reality of the pharmacy practice where community pharmacists have to act as entrepreneurs, and hospital pharmacists are managers staying within drug budgets.

A ninth paper looked at the way in which the industrial pharmacist subsection of the PHAR-QA first round data ranked the fundamental competences for pharmacy practice. As in the two previous papers, European industrial pharmacists (n = 135) ranked 68 competences for practice, arranged into 13 clusters of two types (personal and patient care). The results showed that, compared to community pharmacists (n = 258), industrial pharmacists ranked competences centering on research and development and production of drugs higher, and those centering on patient care lower. Competences centering on values, communication skills, etc. were ranked similarly by the two groups of pharmacists.

In a tenth paper, the results for European students (n = 370) were compared to those for academics (n = 241) and community pharmacists (n = 258). The ranking of the 68 competences by all three groups were similar. This was especially true for the comparison between students and community pharmacists concerning patient care competences, suggesting that students have a good idea of their future profession. A comparison of first and fifth (final) year students showed more awareness of patient care competences in the final year students. Differences did exist, however, between students and community pharmacists. Students—like academics—ranked competences concerned with industrial pharmacy and the quality aspects of preparing drugs, as well as scientific fundamentals of pharmacy practice well above the rankings of community pharmacists. There were no substantial differences amongst the rankings of students from different countries, although some countries have more "medicinal" courses than others. This is, to our knowledge, the first paper to look at how, within a healthcare sectoral profession such as pharmacy, the views on the relative importance of different competences for practice of those educating the future professionals and their students compare to the views of working professionals.

In an eleventh paper, we asked the question as to whether university education influences more than practice the ranking of the importance of competences for practice by community pharmacists coming from different educational backgrounds. We carried out a sub-analysis of the ranking of 68 competences for pharmacy practice in seven countries with different pharmacy education systems in terms of the relative importance of the subject areas of chemical and medicinal sciences. The ranking was very similar in the seven countries, suggesting that the evaluation of competences for practice is based more on the professional experience than on prior university education. There were some differences though, for instance in research-related competence, and these may be influenced by education.

Jeffrey Atkinson
University of Lorraine
Pharmacolor Consultants Nancy
France

pharmacy

MDPI

Concept Paper
Heterogeneity of Pharmacy Education in Europe [†]

Jeffrey Atkinson

Pharmacolor Consultants Nancy, 12 rue de Versigny, Villers 54600, France; jeffrey.atkinson@univ-lorraine.fr; Tel./Fax: +33-383-27-37-03

† This article is dedicated to the memory of Bart Rombaut, co-ordinator of the PHARMINE project, who passed away in January 2014.

Received: 12 June 2014; in revised form: 3 August 2014; Accepted: 11 August 2014; Published: 15 August 2014

Abstract: The 1985 European Economic Community (EEC) directive on the sectoral profession of pharmacy assumed that the comparability of pharmacy education across Europe could provide a basis for the mutual recognition of diplomas. A study by the European Association of Faculties of Pharmacy (EAFP) in 1994 showed, however, that there was large variability in course content. The 2011 PHARMINE study investigated whether such variability had decreased. Information from across the EU countries on the number of contact hours in specific subject areas was compared for the years of 1994 and 2011. Data was obtained from the original 1994 Bourlioux/EAFP study and the 2011 PHARMINE survey. As the latter was based on the 1994 survey, the questions and categories were similar. Results show that there has not been a fall in the variability of course content. Furthermore, EU pharmacy courses have become more "clinical" with an increase in contact hours in the subject area of medicinal sciences.

Keywords: pharmacy; education; clinical; policy; EU

1. Introduction

Pharmacy education and practice in the EU are under the auspices of the directive on sectoral professions that aims at bringing education in line with practice, and ensuring that education throughout the EU is harmonized leading to mutual recognition of diplomas by member states.

The 1985 European Economic Community directive [1] pertained to "the coordination of provisions laid down by law, regulation or administrative action in respect of certain activities in the field of pharmacy" and this " ... with a view to achieving mutual recognition of diplomas". The 1985 directive set out the organizational aspects of pharmacy studies (overall duration, duration of traineeship) and the subject areas of a European pharmacy degree course (see annex), this with a view to fulfilment of the specific activities of a pharmacist in the EU, the latter also set out in the directive.

The 1985 directive stated that "the broad comparability of training courses in the Member States enables coordination in this field to be confined to the requirement that minimum standards be observed, thus leaving the Member States freedom of organization as regards teaching". Thus based on the assumption that courses in Europe were broadly comparable—with little variation in the subject matters treated—recognition of qualifications for sectoral profession of pharmacy could be automatic.

In the early 1990s, the European Association of Faculties of Pharmacy (EAFP) [2] questioned this assumption. P. Bourlioux and others from the EAFP surveyed pharmacy courses in the 11 European Economic Community member states (Belgium, Denmark, France, Germany, Greece, Ireland, Italy, The Netherlands, Portugal, Spain, and the United Kingdom) with pharmacy faculties [3]. They found that although globally the emphasis was on chemical sciences (CHEMSCI), there was wide variation in contact hours in other subjects, for example, medicinal sciences (MEDISCI).

In 2011, the PHARMINE (*PHARMacy Education IN Europe*) EU-funded project [4] in preparation of the 2013 revision of the European directive [5], revisited this problem to see whether the variability in contact hours in specific subject areas had diminished over the previous decades. Using the methodology of the 1994 Bourlioux/EAFP study, the 2011 PHARMINE study gathered data on the contact hours in specific subject areas in the EU member states with pharmacy faculties: the 11 of the 1994 study (see above) plus the 14 countries that had joined the EU at a later date (Austria, Bulgaria, Czech Republic, Estonia, Finland, Hungary, Latvia, Lithuania, Malta, Poland, Rumania, Slovakia, Slovenia, Sweden); the data were revised for this paper with the addition of those for Croatia that joined the EU in 2013.

This paper looks secondly at whether the changes in pharmacy education with a shift towards more clinical activities (an increase in the importance of MEDISCI) correspond to changes in policy (as finalized in the 2013 EU directive).

2. Methods

Information from across the EU countries on the number of contact hours in specific subject areas was compared for the years of 1994 and 2011. Data was obtained from the original 1994 Bourlioux/EAFP study and the 2011 PHARMINE survey, which is described in previous publications. As the latter was based on the 1994 survey, the questions and categories were similar with the main difference being that the PHARMINE survey added a topic on generic subjects.

Data on contact hours in specific subject areas (expressed as a percentage of total hours) for the 1994 Bourlioux/EAFP study were obtained from previous publications [6]. In the 2011 PHARMINE survey [7] an electronic questionnaire was sent out to at least two faculties per country (excepting countries with only one faculty, e.g., Estonia). The departments surveyed in the two studies were not necessarily the same.

Work Programme 1 of the PHARMINE survey centred on the organisation of the activities of pharmacists and professional bodies. It revealed the national background pharmaceutical situation in each member state. Work Programme 2 gathered data on departments, their status (public or private), and their organisation (link to a medical or science faculty …) and on staff and student numbers, entry requirements, courses, and fees. Work Programme 3 looked at data on teaching and learning methods (hours spent on lectures/tutorials/practicals/ independent project work; traineeship; electives). The results of these three work Programmes have been published [8]. Work Programmes 5 and 6 studied the impact of the Bologna declaration and of the EU directive on pharmacy education [9], respectively. Work Programme 6 examined quality assurance in pharmacy education in the EU [10]. (Work Programme 4 dealt with dissemination of the PHARMINE results).

Work Programme 7 looked at the contact hours in specific subject areas shown in the annex. The subject areas were similar in the two studies with the exception of the introduction of a specific chapter for generic subjects in the PHARMINE survey.

The results of Work Programme 7 are presented here with, firstly, separate descriptive analyses of the 1994 and the 2011 studies to determine if there were consistent differences across all countries in the number of hours dedicated to the topic areas. Secondly a comparison of the results of the two studies was carried out to see if there were any differences. Thirdly results from the 2011 PHARMINE study were analysed to see whether the subject area MEDISCI was predominant.

Statistical Analysis

As normality of distributions is unknown for the type of data presented here the Kolmogorov–Smirnov test for deviations of distribution from normality [11] was performed. This showed that only 7%–14% of the data showed significant deviations from normality of distribution (results not shown), thus it was assumed that parametric tests would be robust enough [12].

Results are expressed as means $\pm$ standard deviations, and coefficients of variation (%) = ((mean/standard deviation) $\times$ 100). Comparisons were made using one-way ANOVA followed by the Tukey test for multiple comparisons [13], two-way ANOVA followed by the Holm-Šídák test

Pharmacy **2014**, *2*, 231–243

for multiple comparisons [14], or linear regression ANOVA. Statistical analysis was performed using GraphPad®, [15] programs.

Complete data for each country can be obtained on the PHARMINE website [16]. These profiles were written by the various members of the PHARMINE consortium (see acknowledgements). Data were checked by the author with that available on the department website, where possible.

3. Results

Contact hours in specific subject areas in the 1994 Bourlioux/EAFP and in the 2011 PHARMINE survey (n = 11 countries):

In the 1994 study, subject contact hours were ranked as follows: CHEMSI >> BIOLSCI > MEDISCI > PHARMTECH >> PHYSMATH > LAWSOC (subject areas: Appendix A).

The Tukey test for multiple comparisons showed significant differences ($p < 0.05$) amongst contact hours in subject areas as follows: CHEMSCI greater than the other five; MEDISCI greater than PHYSMATH, PHARMTECH and LAWSOC; and LAWSOC smaller than all others except PHARMTECH. Coefficients of variability were high ranging from 21 to 83% (Table 1).

In the 2011 study, subject contact hours were ranked as follows: MEDISCI > CHEMSI >> PHARMTECH > BIOLSCI >> PHYSMATH > LAWSOC.

The Tukey test for multiple comparisons showed significant differences ($p < 0.05$) amongst contact hours in subject areas as follows: CHEMSCI greater than the other six except MEDISCI; MEDISCI greater than the other six except CHELSCI; and LAWSOC smaller than all others except GENERIC (Table 1). Coefficients of variability were high ranging from 29 to 60%.

Table 1. Contact hours in specific subject areas (expressed as a percentage of total hours) in the 1994 Bourlioux/EAFP and in the 2011 PHARMINE survey (n = 11). See annex for explanation of subject areas.

	CHEMSCI	PHYSMATH	BIOLSCI	PHARMTECH	MEDISCI	LAWSOC
1994						
Mean ± standard deviation	33 ± 7	8 ± 3	21 ± 6	13 ± 5	19 ± 7	6 ± 5
Coefficient of variation (%)	21	38	29	38	37	83
2011						
Mean ± standard deviation	26 ± 11	7 ± 2	13 ± 5	14 ± 5	28 ± 8	5 ± 3
Coefficient of variation (%)	42	29	38	36	29	60

Contact hours in specific subjects in the 2011 PHARMINE survey (n = 26 countries):

Minimum and maximum percentages for CHEMSCI were 14 and 44; for PHYSMATH 2 and 11; for BIOLSCI 2 and 24; for PHARMTECH 6 and 23; for MEDISCI 16 and 42; for LAWSOC 1 and 16; and for GENERIC 1 and 24 (Table 2).

Ranking for mean percentages in subject areas was MEDISCI > CHEMSCI > PHARMTECH > BIOLSCI > GENERIC > PHYSMATH > LAWSOC.

The Tukey test (columns = subject area) showed that there were significant differences in that CHEMSCI was greater than all others except MEDSCI; MEDSCI was greater than all others except CHEMSCI; and that PHARMTECH was greater than PHYSMATH, LAWSOC and GENERIC. Two-way ANOVA (columns = subject area, rows = countries) showed a significant effect of subject areas but not of countries.

There were large coefficients of variation ranging from 25% for MEDSIC to 74% for GENERIC.

Table 2. Contact hours in specific subject areas (expressed as a percentage of total hours) in the 2011 PHARMINE survey (n = 26).

	CHEMSCI	PHYSMATH	BIOLSCI	PHARMTECH	MEDISCI	LAWSOC	GENERIC
Austria	44.0	2.0	22.0	14.0	16.0	0.6	1.0
Belgium	24.0	9.0	11.0	18.0	27.0	2.0	8.0
Bulgaria	31.0	7.0	11.0	13.0	24.0	7.0	7.0
Croatia	24.9	4.2	9.2	8.9	26.9	2.5	23.3
Czech Republic	17.0	5.0	8.0	22.0	19.0	13.0	16.0
Denmark	42.0	7.0	7.0	16.0	16.0	9.0	3.0
Estonia	21.0	4.0	2.0	21.0	39.0	10.0	3.0
Finland	20.0	5.6	2.5	21.9	28.8	15.6	5.6
France	17.6	9.5	17.9	5.9	42.0	2.2	5.0
Germany	39.8	4.5	10.9	13.4	28.3	2.1	3.8
Greece	39.3	5.8	14.2	8.2	15.9	2.7	14.0
Hungary	27.2	5.2	5.2	16.0	28.5	3.9	14.2
Ireland	13.6	11.1	7.1	18.3	35.5	7.3	7.1
Italy	32.4	7.2	10.4	9.1	31.5	4.8	2.2
Latvia	27.7	6.4	6.4	20.2	26.6	8.5	6.4
Lithuania	21.3	2.0	8.9	8.9	27.7	7.4	23.8
Malta	15.4	7.2	12.7	15.4	30.8	3.6	15.0
Netherlands	20.1	3.9	10.6	14.2	31.1	8.3	11.8
Poland	21.3	4.1	8.0	15.9	38.2	6.2	6.2
Portugal	19.6	6.8	14.6	14.9	32.2	12.0	1.2
Rumania	26.1	8.7	15.8	14.1	24.9	3.7	6.6
Slovakia	28.8	8.8	10.9	14.4	27.6	3.4	6.0
Slovenia	27.0	8.5	8.5	22.0	21.0	8.5	4.7
Spain	23.5	5.5	19.9	11.0	27.6	5.5	7.0
Sweden	18.3	11.3	12.8	19.5	21.5	11.8	5.0
United Kingdom	13.6	5.7	23.9	22.7	23.9	3.4	6.8
Mean	25.3	6.4	11.2	15.3	27.4	6.3	8.2
Standard deviation	8.6	2.5	5.4	4.8	6.8	3.9	6.1
Coefficient of variation (%)	33.9	38.4	48.5	31.2	25.0	61.8	74.3

There was a significant inverse linear relationship between MEDSCI and CHEMSCI (CHEMSCI = $-0.61 \times$ MEDSCI $+ 43$, $R^2 = 0.26$, $p < 0.05$); Figure 1.

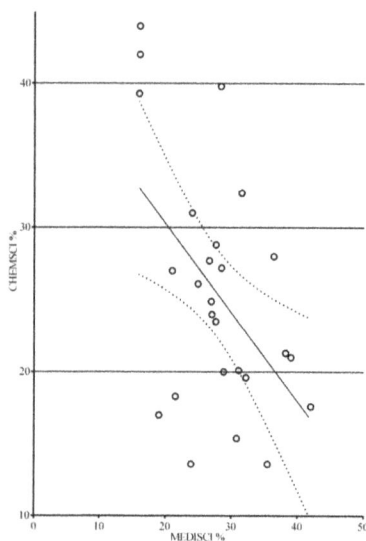

Figure 1. Linear relationship between MEDISCI and CHEMSCI (n = 26 countries).

4. Discussion

4.1. Methodology.

In both surveys all the participants were members of the EAFP. Thus this study does not involve randomly drawn departments. In addition the departments surveyed in the second study were not necessarily the same as those surveyed in the first. The impact of this on results is unknown. In 1994 the European Economic Community was composed of a small number of member states most with a large population (> 10,000,000): Belgium, France, Germany, Greece, Italy, The Netherlands, Portugal, Spain, and the United Kingdom. In 2014 the EU has more than doubled in size as many countries with smaller populations have joined. In larger countries there are several pharmacy departments (> 20 in France, Germany, Spain and the UK) and national bodies fix courses. In smaller countries there may be only one or two departments and these tend to look more towards EU organisations for guidance on courses. Thus the contexts of the 1994 Bourlioux survey and of the PHARMINE survey are different. Finally, Scotland represented the UK in the 1994 Bourlioux/EAFP survey, whereas as England represented the UK in the PHARMINE study. Organisation of pharmacy education in the two countries is not identical but similar. In most cases each member state was represented by data from a single department, in a few cases by two departments. There was no attempt to survey a number of departments relative to the size of the country.

The organisation of the subject areas used in the 2011 PHARMINE study was that used by the 1994 Bourlioux/EAFP survey, the latter being based on the EEC 1985 directive (see Appendix A). This allows comparison between the two studies and evaluation of possible evolution. However, other patterns of organisation are possible. In some faculties of pharmacy, "Pharmaceutical Sciences" contains the core subject areas in pharmaceutical education and research. This encompasses pharmaceutical technology, pharmacological sciences (including pharmacology–basic and clinical–pharmacokinetics, pharmacotherapy, toxicology, *i.e.*, all drug action and use-related subjects such as medical devices, drugs in veterinary medicine, *etc.*) and social pharmacy. All the other subjects pertain strictly speaking to biomedical sciences and are grouped in what is called "Medicinal Sciences". In other words anatomy, physiology, *etc.* are in fact "Biomedical Sciences" (not "Biomedicinal") and the drug-related subjects (even though they are included in medicinal sciences) are within "Pharmacological Sciences". In particular, for example radiochemistry may be included in CHEMSCI and pharmaceutical care in LAWSOC.

Finally, there are also organisational differences between the EU directive 2013/55 and modern-day pharmacy education and practice. Thus, for example, clinical chemistry (or clinical biology) exists as an area of pharmacy practice and education in many member states but is not included in EU directive 2013/55.

4.2. Evolution in Subject Areas between the 1994 and 2011 Surveys

Percentages for PHYSMATH, BIOLSCI and PHARMTECH showed little change. CHEMSCI decreased from 33% to 26%, that for BIOLSCI from 21% to 13%, and that for MEDSCI increased from 19% to 28%.

The coefficients of variation for means of hours in subject areas were similar in the two surveys. Thus the variability between member states has not decreased since the 1990s in spite of the staff and student exchange between countries via the Erasmus [17] and other programmes, and course harmonization tools such as the European Credit Transfer and Accumulation System (ECTS) [18].

It could be argued that the differences (variability) among the pharmacy curricula are not necessarily negative. Variability in educational procedures can be useful as it allows academic freedom to try other approaches, and prevents departments from all making the same mistake.

Finally it remains to be seen if variability in pharmacy curricula is really producing significant variability in pharmacists' competences for practice.

4.3. A More "Clinical" Education and Practice in Pharmacy?

There is a shift in pharmacy education over the previous decades from courses oriented towards CHEMSCI to those oriented towards MEDSCI. In the 1994 study MEDISCI was ranked third in number of contact hours, far behind CHEMSCI, whereas in the 2011 study MEDISCI was ranked first.

The above change in pharmacy education to more "clinical" courses is in line with the main changes in the directive between 1985 and 2013 and the inclusion of notions of:

(1) safe and efficacious medicinal products
(2) provision of information and advice on medicinal products . . . including on their appropriate use
(3) reporting of adverse reactions of pharmaceutical products
(4) provision of personalised support for patients
(5) contribution to local or national public health campaigns

Thus the list of specific activities of a pharmacist given in the 1985/432/EEC directive has been extended by additions (in bold below) in the 2013/55/EU directive:

(a) preparation of the pharmaceutical form of medicinal products
(b) manufacture and testing of medicinal products
(c) testing of medicinal products in a laboratory for the testing of medicinal products
(d) storage, preservation and distribution of medicinal products at the wholesale stage
(e) supply, preparation, testing, storage, **distribution and dispensing of safe and efficacious medicinal products of the required quality** in pharmacies open to the public
(f) preparation, testing, storage and dispensing of **safe and efficacious medicinal products of the required quality** in hospitals
(g) provision of information and advice on medicinal products **as such, including on their appropriate use**
(h) **reporting of adverse reactions of pharmaceutical products to the competent authorities**
(i) **personalised support for patients who administer their medication**
(j) **contribution to local or national public health campaigns**

The above changes in the directive underlie a shift in the practice of pharmacy towards a more "clinical" role with involvement of more MEDISCI elements. This ties in with the trend towards courses with a higher MEDISCI percentage noted above.

Albeit, the linear relationship between CHEMSCI and MEDISCI (Figure 1) reveals that there are exceptions with some countries (e.g., Austria, Denmark, Germany) giving more "chemical" courses as judged from the relative hours dedicated to CHEMSCI and MEDISCI. This inverse relationship also shows that alongside countries like Poland, Estonia and France with a more "clinical" course, there are countries like Romania, Hungary and Slovenia with a "balanced" curriculum.

The change to a more "clinical" approach is not a uniquely EU phenomenon as judged by the increase world-wide in the number of publications on, for example, "pharmaceutical care" from 1 in 1990 to 104 in 2011, with 50 citations to articles on pharmaceutical care in 1995, and 1300 in 2011.

5. Conclusions

The conclusions to this study are:

- Since the 1990s there has been no decrease in the variability in pharmacy courses amongst departments in different countries. This raises the question of the difference between the notion of *"the broad comparability of training courses in the Member States"* as outlined in the 1985 EEC directive, and the reality of the variability of EU pharmacy education systems.

- In the EU, there has been a shift towards more "clinical" courses with a greater MEDISCI content. This global shift from courses oriented towards chemical sciences to those oriented towards medicinal sciences coincides with the recognition—in the latest version of the EU directive—of a more important "clinical" role for pharmacists.

Appendix A

Table A1. Subject areas in the 1985 EEC directive together with additions in 1994 Bourlioux/EAFP survey (non-italic) and in the 2011 PHARMINE survey (italic).

Subject Areas in Directive 85/432/EEC	Additional Subjects
1. Chemistry (CHEMSCI)	
General and inorganic chemistry Organic chemistry Analytical chemistry Pharmaceutical chemistry including analysis of medicinal products	Medical physico-chemistry Pharmacopeia analysis
	Structure-activity relationships / drug design
2. Physics / Mathematics / Computing / Statistics (PHYSMATH)	
Physics	Mathematics / Computing / Statistics *Pharmaceutical calculations* *Information technology, information technology applied to community pharmacy, information technology applied to national healthcare* *Experimental design and analysis*
3. Biology / Biochemistry / Pharmacognosy (BIOLSCI)	
General and applied biochemistry (medical) Plant and animal biology Microbiology/Pharmacognosy	Phyto-chemistry
	Mycology *Molecular biology* *Genetics*
4. Pharmaceutics / Technology (PHARMTECH)	
Pharmaceutical technology	Finished medicinal products
	Drug disposition and metabolism / pharmacokinetics
	Novel drug delivery systems
	Pharmaceutical research and development
	Drug production
	Quality assurance in production
	Drug / new chemical entity registration and regularization Common technical document: pharmaceutical quality, safety pharmacology and toxicology efficacy (preclinical and clinical studies) Ophthalmic preparations
	Medical gases
	Cosmetics
	Management strategy in industry Economics of the pharmaceutical industry and of research and development

Table A1. *Cont.*

Subject Areas in Directive 85/432/EEC	Additional Subjects
5. Medicine / Pharmacology / Toxicology (MEDISCI)	
Anatomy, physiology, medical terminology	*Pathology / Histology / Nutrition*
Pharmacology / pharmacotherapy Toxicology	*Haematology / Immunology Parasitology / Hygiene Emergency therapy*
	Non-pharmacological treatment Clinical chemistry / bio-analysis (of body fluids) Radiochemistry
	Dispensing process, drug prescription, prescription analysis (detection of adverse effects and drug interactions)
	Generic drugs Planning, running and interpretation of the data of clinical trials Medical devices Orthopaedics OTC medicines, complementary therapy At-home support and care Skin illness and treatment Homeopathy Phyto-therapy Drugs in veterinary medicine Pharmaceutical care, pharmaceutical therapy of illness and disease
6. Law / Social Aspects of Pharmacy (LAWSOC)	
Legislation / professional ethics	Philosophy / Economics
	Management / History of pharmacy
	Public health
	Social sciences Forensic science Public health / health promotion Quality management Epidemiology of drug use (pharmaco-epidemiology) Economics of drug use (pharmaco-economics)
7.Generic Competences (GENERIC)	
	General knowledge
	Academic literacy Languages First aid Communication Management Practical skills

Acknowledgments: The author thanks the following persons who provided the raw data:

C. Noe. University of Vienna. Austria.
B. Rombaut. H. Halewijck and B. Thys. Vrije Universiteit Brussel. Faculty of Medicine and Pharmacy. Dept. Pharmaceutical Biotechnology and Molecular Biology. Brussels. Belgium.
V. Petkova and S. Nikolov. University of Sofia. Faculty of Pharmacy. Sofia. Bulgaria.
V. Belcheva. Sanofi-Aventis. Sofia. Bulgaria.
M. Z. Končić. University of Zagreb. Faculty of Pharmacy and Biochemistry. Zagreb Croatia.
D. Jonjic. Croatian Chamber of Pharmacists. Zagreb. Croatia.
Crnkovic. Hospital pharmacy. Psychiatry Clinic. Zagreb. Croatia.
M. Polasek. Faculty of Pharmacy. Charles University. Prague. Czech Republic.
U. Madsen and B. Fjalland. Faculty of Pharmaceutical Sciences. University of Copenhagen. Denmark.
M. Brandl. Faculty of Science. University of Southern Denmark. Denmark.
M. Ringkjøbing-Elema. EIPG / The Association of Danish Industrial Pharmacists. Copenhagen. Denmark.
P. Veski and D. Volmer. Department of Pharmacy. University of Tartu. Tartu. Estonia.
J. Hirvonen and A. Juppo. University of Helsinki. Faculty of Pharmacy. Finland.
Capdeville-Atkinson. Lorraine University. Nancy. France.
Marcincal. Faculté de Pharmacie. Université de Lille 2. Lille. France.
V. Lacamoire and I. Baron. Conseil National de l'Ordre des Pharmaciens. Paris. France.
R. Süss and R. Schubert. University of Freiburg. Freiburg. Germany.
P. Macheras. E. Mikros and D. M. Rekkas. School of Pharmacy. University of Athens. Athens. Greece.
K. Poulas. School of Pharmacy. University of Patras. Patras. Greece.

Pharmacy **2014**, *2*, 231–243

G. Soos and P. Doro. Faculty of Pharmacy. University of Szeged. Szeged. Hungary.
J. Strawbridge and P. Gallagher. Royal College of Surgeons in Ireland. Dublin. Ireland.
L. Horgan. Pharmaceutical Society of Ireland. PSI—The Pharmacy Regulator. Dublin. Ireland.
Rossi. and P. BLASI Faculty of Pharmacy. University of Perugia. Perugia. Italy.
R. Muceniece. Faculty of Medicine of University of Latvia. Riga. Latvia.
Maurina. Faculty of Pharmacy. Riga. Latvia.
Saprovska. Latvian Branch. European Industrial Pharmacists' Group (EIPG). Riga. Latvia.
V. Briedis and M. Sapragoniene. Lithuanian University of Health Sciences. Kaunus. Lithuania.
L. M. Azzopardi and A. S. Inglott. University of Malta. Department of Pharmacy. Msida. Malta.
T. Schalekamp. Utrecht University. Faculty of Science. Department of Pharmaceutical Sciences. Utrecht. The Netherlands.
H. J. Haisma. University of Groningen. School of Life Sciences. Pharmacy and Pharmaceutical Sciences. Groningen. The Netherlands.
S. Polak and R. Jachowicz. Faculty of Pharmacy with Division of Medicinal Analysis. Jagiellonian University Medical College. Krakow. Poland.
J. A. G. Morais and A.M. Cavaco. Faculdade de Farmácia Universidade de Lisboa. Lisbon. Portugal.
Mircioiu and C. Rais. Faculty of Pharmacy. University of Medicine and Pharmacy "Carol Davila". Bucharest. Romania.
J. Kyselovič and M. Remko. Faculty of Pharmacy. Comenius University. Odbojarov 10. Bratislava. 83232. Slovakia.
Bozic and S. Gobec. University of Ljubljana. Faculty of Pharmacy. Ljubljana. Slovenia.
B. DEL Castillo-Garcia. Facultad de Farmacia. Universidad Complutense de Madrid. Madrid. Spain.
L. Recalde and A. Sanchez Pozo. Facultad de Farmacia. Universidad de Granada. Granada. Spain.
R. Hansson and E. Björk. Faculty of Pharmacy. Uppsala University; G. TOBIN. Sahlgrenska Academy. Sweden.
K. A Wilson. Aston Pharmacy School. Aston. UK.
G. B. Lockwood. University of Manchester. School of Pharmacy. Manchester. UK.

The opinions expressed in this paper are those of its author.

Conflicts of Interest: The author declares no conflict of interest.

References

1. Council Directive of 16 September 1985 concerning the coordination of provisions laid down by law, regulation or administrative action in respect of certain activities in the field of pharmacy. Available online: http://eur-lex.europa.eu/legal-content/EN/TXT/PDF/?uri=CELEX:31985L0432&from=EN (accessed on 23 July 2014).

2. European Association of Faculties of Pharmacy (EAFP). Available online: http://eafponline.eu/ (accessed on 3 August 2014).

3. ERASMUS Subject Evaluations: Summary Reports of the Evaluation Conferences by Subject Area. *pharmacy*. volume 1. Available online: http://ec.europa.eu/education/erasmus/doc/publ/conf_en.pdf (accessed on 23 July 2014).

4. PHARMINE: pharmacy education in Europe. Available online: http://www.pharmine.org/ (accessed on 23 July 2014).

5. EU directive 2013/55/EU on the recognition of professional qualifications. Available online: http://eur-lex.europa.eu/LexUriServ/LexUriServ.do?uri=OJ:L:2005:255:0022:0142:EN:PDF (accessed on 23 July 2014).

6. Bourlioux, P. Proceedings of the 2nd European meetings of the faculties, schools and institutes of pharmacy. Berlin, September 1994; Available online: http://enzu.pharmine.org/media/filebook/files/Bourlioux_full_report.pdf (accessed on 23 July 2014).

7. The PHARMINE WP7 survey. Available online: http://enzu.pharmine.org/media/filebook/files/PHARMINE%20WP7%20survey%20of%20European%20HEIs%200309.pdf (accessed on 23 July 2014).

8. Atkinson, J; Rombaut, B. The 2011 PHARMINE report on pharmacy and pharmacy education in the European Union. *Pharm. Pract.* **2011**, *9*, 169–187.

9. Atkinson, J,; Rombaut, B. The PHARMINE study on the impact of the European Union directive on sectoral professions and of the Bologna declaration on pharmacy education in Europe. *Pharm. Pract.* **2011**, *9*, 188–194.

10. Guimarães Morais, J.A.; Cavaco, A.M.; Rombaut, B.; Rouse, M.; Atkinson, J. Quality assurance in European pharmacy education and training. *Pharm. Pract.* **2011**, *9*, 195–199.

Pharmacy **2014**, *2*, 231–243

11. Kolmogorov–Smirnov test for deviations of distribution from normality. Available online: http://www. graphpad.com/www/data-analysis-resource-center/blog/new-in-prism-6-kolmogorov-smirnov-test/ (accessed on 3 August 2014).
12. Raschi, D.; Guiard, V. The robustness of parametric statistical methods. *Psychol. Sci.* **2004**, *4*, 175–208.
13. Tukey test for multiple comparisons. Available online: http://www.graphpad.com/guides/prism/6/ statistics/index.htm?stat_the_methods_of_tukey_and_dunne.htm (accessed on 3 August 2014).
14. Holm-Šídák test for multiple comparisons. Available online: http://www.graphpad.com/guides/prism/6/ statistics/index.htm?stat_holms_multiple_comparison_test.htm (accessed on 3 August 2014).
15. GraphPad®. Available online: http://www.graphpad.com/ (accessed on 23 July 2014).
16. Country profiles on the PHARMINE website. Available online: http://www.pharmine.org/losse_paginas/ Country_Profiles/ (accessed on 23 July 2014).
17. Erasmus. Available online: https://www.erasmusplus.org.uk/ (accessed on 3 August 2014).
18. European Credit Transfer and Accumulation System (ECTS). Available online: http://ec.europa.eu/ education/tools/docs/ects-guide_en.pdf (accessed on 23 July 2014).

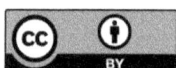

pharmacy

MDPI

Review

Systems for Quality Assurance in Pharmacy Education and Training in the European Union

Jeffrey Atkinson [1],*, Bart Rombaut [2], Antonio Sánchez Pozo [3], Dimitrios Rekkas [4], Peep Veski [5], Jouni Hirvonen [6], Borut Bozic [7], Agnieska Skowron [8], Constantin Mircioiu [9], Annie Marcincal [10] and Keith Wilson [11]

[1] Pharmacology Department Lorraine University, Pharmacolor Consultants Nancy, 12 rue de Versigny, Villers 54600, France

[2] European Association of Faculties of Pharmacy (EAFP), Vrije Universiteit Brussel (VUB), Laarbeeklaan 103, Brussels 1090, Belgium; brombaut@vub.ac.be

[3] Faculty of Pharmacy, University of Granada (UGR), Campus Universitario de la Cartuja s/n, Granada 18701, Spain; sanchezpster@gmail.com

[4] School of Pharmacy, National and Kapodistrian University Athens, (UoA), Panepistimiou 30, Athens 10679, Greece; rekkas@pharm.uoa.gr

[5] Pharmacy Faculty, University of Tartu (UT), Nooruse 1, Tartu 50411, Estonia; peep.veski@ut.ee

[6] Pharmacy Faculty, University of Helsinki (UH), Yliopistonkatu 4, P.O. Box 33-4, Helsinki 00014, Finland; jouni.hirvonen@helsinki.fi

[7] Faculty of Pharmacy, University of Ljubjana (ULFFA), Askerceva cesta 7, Ljubljana 1000, Slovenia; Borut.Bozic@ffa.uni-lj.si

[8] Pharmacy Faculty, Jagiellonian University (JUMC), UL. Golebia 24, Krakow 31-007, Poland; askowron@cm-uj.krakow.pl

[9] Pharmacy Faculty, University of Medicine and Pharmacy "Carol Davila" Bucharest (UMFCD-B), Dionisie Lupu 37, Bucharest 020021, Romania; constantin.mircioiu@yahoo.com

[10] Université de Lille 2 (UL), Lille 59000, France; annie.marcincal@pharma.univ-lille2.fr

[11] School of Life and Health Sciences, Aston University (AU), Birmingham, B4 7ET, England; k.a.wilson@aston.ac.uk

* Author to whom correspondence should be addressed; jeffrey.atkinson@univ-lorraine.fr; Tel.: +33-383-27-37-03; Fax. +33-383-27-37-03.

Received: 17 October 2013; in revised form: 12 December 2013; Accepted: 13 December 2013; Published: 2 January 2014

Abstract: With the changes in the Bologna process and the European directive on sectoral professions, the education and training of the pharmacists in the European Higher Education Area is moving towards a quality system based on competences. In this paper we analyze the existing quality assurance and accreditation systems in 10 countries and examine how far these systems have evolved from a resources and curriculum basis towards a competences basis. This is the first step towards the goal of the PHAR-QA project: establishment of a European quality assurance system based on competences. Existing systems of quality assurance for pharmacy education and teaching are based mainly on resources and management not competences. Furthermore, they are national, obligatory, and do not recognize all the current activities of the pharmacists. The PHAR-QA system that will be developed by the consortium of the same name will be based on competences; it will be European, consultative, and will encompass pharmacy practice in a wide sense.

Keywords: pharmacy; education; quality assurance; competences

1. Introduction

The establishment of the European Higher Education Area has led universities to harmonize and modernize their educational systems in order to increase mutual recognition needed for student and citizen mobility. The Bologna process is moving from programs based on content and class hours towards programs based on competences [1]. The use of competences and credits leads to harmonization of programs eliminating ambiguity in syllabi and clearly establishing what the student—at the end of the program—is able to do.

All EU pharmacy degree programs follow the European Directive 2005/36 for the recognition of qualifications for sectoral professions and are basically described in terms of content. The definition of the programs in terms of competences is becoming necessary not only because of the changes in the Bologna process, but also because of changes in the role of the pharmacist as defined in the new amendment to the EU directive (see below).

In this paper, we describe the quality assurance and accreditation systems in 10 different countries.

There are several constraints on pharmacy education and training in the European Union that necessitate the development of a new quality assurance system. The reasons for the need for a new system stem from the different points below:

1.1. EU Directive on Sectoral Professions

The shortly to be amended [2] EU directive on sectoral professions 2005/36/EC [3] deals with the management (5-year course duration with 6-month training period during or at the end of the course), and knowledge and skills (the word "competence" is not used) required in pharmacy education and training.

Knowledge and skills are developed as follows:

Pharmacy **2014**, *2*, 17–26

Box 1

Course subjects (Annex V.6, 5.61)

(1)   Plant and animal biology
(2)   Physics
(3)   General and inorganic chemistry
(4)   Organic chemistry
(5)   Analytical chemistry
(6)   Pharmaceutical chemistry, including analysis of medicinal products
(7)   and applied biochemistry (medical)
(8)   General and physiology; medical terminology
(9)   Microbiology
(10)   Pharmacology and pharmacotherapy
(11)   Pharmaceutical technology
(12)   Toxicology
(13)   Pharmacognosy
(14)   Legislation and, where appropriate, professional ethics.

Knowledge and skills (Article 44.3 of the directive)

(1)   Adequate knowledge of medicines and the substances used in the manufacture of medicines;
(2)   Adequate knowledge of pharmaceutical technology and the physical, chemical, biological and microbiological testing of medicinal products;
(3)   Adequate knowledge of the metabolism and the effects of medicinal products and of the action of toxic substances, and of the use of medicinal products;
(4)   Adequate knowledge to evaluate scientific data concerning medicines in order to be able to supply appropriate information on the basis of this knowledge;
(5)   Adequate knowledge of the legal and other requirements associated with the pursuit of pharmacy.

1.2. The European Higher Education Area

The European Higher Education Area ensures more comparable, compatible and coherent systems of higher education in Europe, building on the principles announced in the Bologna declaration [4]. The latter was signed by 29 European countries and is a collection of recommendations, not a directive. One of the Bologna principles recommends that the degree structure be based on a 3-year bachelor followed by a 2-year master degree, with entry and exit possible at the end of the 3-year bachelor degree. With vary rare exceptions this is not possible in pharmacy education; most countries have a 5-year integrated course. Some countries (e.g., Belgium) have an "academic" bachelor in pharmacy that leads automatically to a master in pharmacy.

1.3. The Diversity of Jobs for Graduates with a Degree in Pharmacy

Most graduates with a degree in pharmacy take up a career in community pharmacy. The European directive on sectoral professions (above) reflects this situation in defining the knowledge and skills required for such practice. The directive does however recognize the existence of hospital pharmacy practice (article 45, Section 2.f of the directive). However, other activities (pharmaceutical industry, pharmaceutical distribution, para-pharmacy, regulatory affairs, laboratory medicine/clinical biology …) are not mentioned in the directive.

1.4. The Evolution in Healthcare

Socio-economic changes in healthcare systems are redefining the role of the pharmacist. This is recognized in the proposed amendment to the directive (see [2]) in which the following additions are made:

- Monitoring of medicinal treatments
- Provision of information and advice on health-related issues in cooperation with medical practitioners
- Reporting of adverse reactions of pharmaceutical products
- Personalized support for patients who administer their own medication
- Contribution to institutional public health campaigns

1.5. The Evolution in the Pharmaceutical Industry

The pharmaceutical industry has undergone changes in its science (switch to biotechnology, development of therapies for unfulfilled needs like Alzheimer's disease, *etc.*) and in its economic structure (interactions between universities and start-ups, development of global multinationals, *etc.*).

It should be noted that the situation regarding points c, d and e above may be different from one country to another.

Any system of pharmacy education and training—and the accompanying quality assurance system—should reply intrinsically to the first constraint above but not neglect the four others.

This constitutes the vision for pharmacy practice in Europe.

2. Methods

In order to perform a cross-sectional analysis of existing European systems, a questionnaire was sent to the first 10 authors of this report who are partners in the PHAR-QA ("Quality Assurance in European pharmacy education and training") consortium. This project is financed by the Education, Audio-visual and Culture Executive Agency [5] (EACEA reference 527194-LLP-1-2012-1-BE-ERASMUS-EMCR). The 11th author in the list is a member of the advisory board.

3. Results and Discussion

3.1. Existing Quality Assurance Systems in Pharmacy Education and Training in 10 Countries of the European Union I agree

The quality assurance systems in the 10 countries studied showed high variability; it is thus impossible to establish a simple, harmonized pattern.

The main elements of the quality assurance systems are given in Table 1.

Table 1. The basis and organization of quality assurance systems in 10 EU pharmacy departments.

Country	Quality assurance system
Belgium	Basis: The auditors check that the university has the resources, structure and management required to ensure that students can acquire adequate competences (generic and pharmaceutical). Organization: Flanders has a cross-border agency that deals with Flanders and The Netherlands [6]. In Wallonia the regional *"Agence pour l'Evaluation de la Qualité de l'Enseignement Supérieur"* [7] handles quality assurance and accreditation, albeit the criteria are the same. There is an audit every seven years (shortly to be changed to five years).
Spain	Basis: Evaluation is essentially based on material and human resources together with other elements such as output, results, and an element of appraisal of competences using the European Qualifications Framework. The main reference level descriptors are: skills, competences and knowledge [8]. Organization: Verification and accreditation are done by the national agency ("The National Agency for Quality Assessment and Accreditation of Spain" [9]); in some autonomous regions this task is delegated to a regional agency. To achieve the accreditation and to renew it (every 6 years), evaluation reports have to be presented according to the specific quality assurance system.
Greece	Basis: The major criteria for assessing quality fall into four categories: curriculum, teaching, research and other services. Organization: The "Hellenic Quality Assurance Agency for Higher Education (HQAA)" [10] is responsible.
Estonia	Basis: Evaluation is based mainly on resources. All activities described are evaluated in terms of finances available and the competences of teaching staff. Organization: The study program in pharmacy is designed, developed and evaluated by the university of Tartu program council. The latter consists of the representatives of professional organizations, staff members from other departments and students. The program manager—currently the head of the pharmacy department—is appointed by the university senate. The program manager and council perform an internal evaluation every 3 years. The tools for self-evaluation are developed by the "Estonian Higher Education Quality Agency" [11] and adapted by the university. In addition student organizations undertake an annual official evaluation of the quality of teaching and the competences of the teaching staff.
Finland	Basis: The system is based on management and competences. Competences are not "pharmacy-specific". Organization: The evaluation system is based on national criteria and executed following the advice and under the supervision of the "Finnish Higher Education Evaluation System (FINHEEC)" [12]. The same principles are applied to all disciplines. Universities develop their own individual systems which are based on FINHEEC standards. Quality assurance systems are audited every 6 years by external examiners nominated by FINHEEC.
Slovenia	Basis: This is essentially on resources. The M. Pharm. program is designed on program structure and partially on needed competences. Organization: The system is national: accreditations of the university and of the program are done by the "Slovenian Quality Assurance Agency for Higher Education" [13]. The system is the same for all programs. Student evaluation is mandatory. Accreditation occurs every 7 years and is based on (a) fulfillment of initial criteria; (b) annual reports for courses; (c) achievement of students' competences; and (d) students' surveys of programs, teacher-student interaction, and courses.
Poland	Basis: The quality criteria are: (1) mission, planning and evaluation; (2) organization and administration; (3) curriculum; (4) student and academic policies; (5) staff resources; and (6) facilities and resources—buildings, scientific equipment, financial resources. Generic competencies for all medical specializations are established as well as specific competences for pharmacy. Organization: The accreditation system is national [14]; the same criteria are used for all universities. Each university has to prepare an accreditation report, which is assessed by an expert panel with independent scientists and experienced academic teachers.

Table 1. *Cont.*

Country	Quality assurance system
Romania	Basis: The evaluation system is based on resources, structures, finances and management. It is not based on competences. The main areas are: institutional capacity, and educational effectiveness. Within the latter, quality assurance strategies and procedures are evaluated. Organization: Verification and accreditation are done by the "National Romanian Agency for Quality Assurance in Higher Education" [15].
France	Basis. The system is based essentially on resources and management. Organization: Quality assurance and accreditation are carried out every five years by the independent "French Evaluation Agency for Research and Higher Education—AERES" [16]. The AERES board is made up of 25 French, European or international members appointed by decree. The curriculum is set by the French Ministry of Education and the organization of courses and examinations is validated by the university council taking into account the proposals of the faculty council. Internal quality assurance systems are run by certain universities.
UK	Basis: There are 10 standards, some concerned with the process and two with the curriculum and the outcomes. Standard 10 is a series of grouped educational outcomes. They are expressed as outcomes rather than competences. Organization: In the UK the "Quality Assurance Agency for Higher Education" [17,18] sets standards for universities. Pharmacy is regulated by the "General Pharmaceutical Council" [19,20], an organization set up by statute and with statutory powers but which is independent of government. The Council sets standards for pharmacy and pharmacy technician education and has powers both for pre-registration education and post-registration (the latter currently only used for independent pharmacy prescribers). The council organizes an accreditation of schools of pharmacy. The council sets the 10 standards for the education of pharmacists that cover the university course and the associated one year pre-registration program.

As a summary of the above table, the system used in most European countries is shown in the diagram (Figure 1).

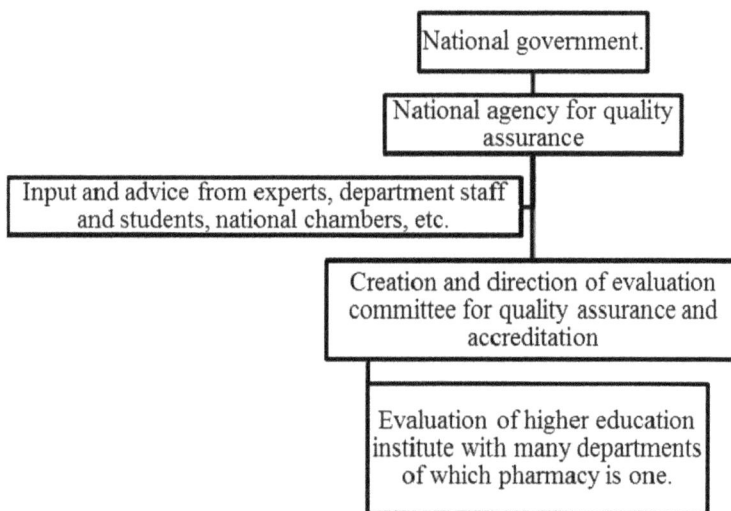

Figure 1. The organization of the national quality assurance system in 10 EU pharmacy departments.

The characteristics of the above system are given in the left-hand column of Table 2.

Table 2. A comparison of national quality assurance systems with that proposed by the PHAR-QA consortium.

National quality assurance system.	PHAR-QA system.
National	European
Based mainly on resources and management	Based on competences
Obligatory	Consultative
Adapted to national economics and politics in matters such as healthcare and pharmaceutical industry	Adapted to European economics and politics in matters such as healthcare and pharmaceutical industry
Reviews and applies to a higher educational institution to which a pharmacy department belongs.	Reviews and applies to a pharmacy department
Periodic: 3–7 year period depending on country	On demand
Applies essentially to public institutions	Applies to all institutions both public and private

In the right-hand column are the characteristics of the proposed PHAR-QA system; this is shown in Figure 2.

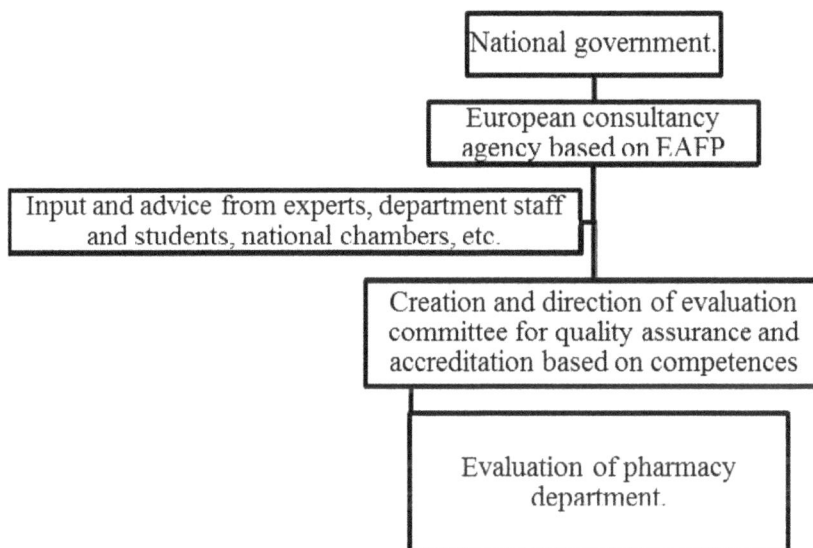

Figure 2. The PHAR-QA project: development of a European quality assurance system based on a competence framework.

3.2. Towards a Pan-European System for Quality Assurance in Pharmacy Education and Training Based on Competences I agree

Our study reveals that the use of competences for quality systems is infrequent.

In the UK, competences for pharmacists have been developed by the "Competency Development and Evaluation Group (CoDEG)" [21] a collaborative network of specialist and academic pharmacists, developers, researchers and practitioners. CoDEG has proposed a "General Level Framework" with competences in patient care, problem solving and management.

A very similar approach was used by the PHARMINE ("Pharmacy education and training in Europe") network that was funded by the EU [22]. PHARMINE work program 3 was directed by Ian Bates who holds the Chair of Pharmacy Education at the University College London School of Pharmacy, and is Head of Educational Development. The competences his group proposed are available on-line at the PHARMINE website.

The PHAR-QA [23] "Quality assurance in European pharmacy education and training" project follows on from PHARMINE. It is also funded by the EU. PHAR-QA will operate according to the schema shown in Figure 3. Validation and refinement will be done using the Delphi method.

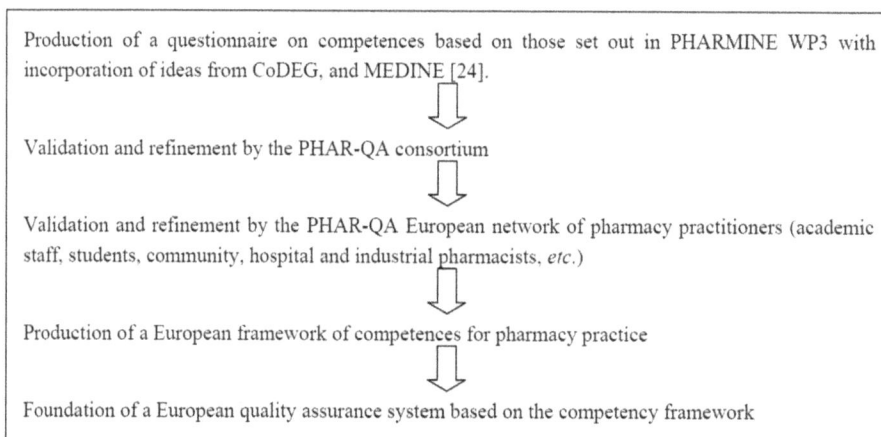

Figure 3. The PHAR-QA "Quality assurance in European pharmacy education and training" project.

4. Conclusions

A review of existing systems of quality assurance for pharmacy education and teaching shows that these are national, obligatory, based mainly on resources and management rather than competences, and adapted to national economics and politics in matters such as healthcare and pharmaceutical industry.

A new system based on competences is required. This is the aim of the PHAR-QA project that will develop a system that is European, consultative, based on competences and adapted to European economics and politics in matters such as healthcare and pharmaceutical industry.

Acknowledgments: PHAR-QA is funded by the European, Education, Audio-visual and Culture Agency (EACEA: eacea.ec.europa.eu/); the grant number is 527194-LLP-1-2012-1-BE-ERASMUS-EMCR.

Conflicts of Interest: The authors declare no conflict of interest.

References

1. Towards Shared Descriptors for Bachelors and Masters. Available online: http://www.ehea.info/article-details.aspx?ArticleId=110 (accessed on 2 December 2013).
2. Vergnaud, B. Proposal for a Directive of the European Parliament and of the Council Amending Directive 2005/36/EC on the Recognition of Professional Qualifications and Regulation on Administrative Cooperation through the Internal Market Information System. Available online: http://www.europarl.europa.eu/meetdocs/2009_2014/documents/imco/dv/vergnaud_profqual_finalreport_/vergnaud_profqual_finalreport_en.pdf (accessed on 2 December 2013).
3. Directive 2005/36/ec of the European Parliament and of the Council of 7 September 2005 on the Recognition of Professional Qualifications. Available online: http://eur-lex.europa.eu/LexUriServ/LexUriServ.do?uri=OJ:L:2005:255:0022:0142:en:PDF (accessed on 2 December 2013).
4. The European Higher Education Area. Available online: http://www.ehea.info/ (accessed on 2 Decembe 2013).

5. Education, Audio-visual and Culture Executive Agency. Available online: http://eacea.ec.europa.eu/index_en.php (accessed on 2 December 2013).

6. The Accreditation Organization of the Netherlands and Flanders. Available online: http://www.nvao.net/ (accessed on 2 December 2013).

7. Agence pour l'Evaluation de la Qualité de l'Enseignement Supérieur. Available online: http://www.aeqes.be/ (accessed on 2 December 2013).

8. European Qualifications Framework. Available online: http://ec.europa.eu/education/lifelong-learning-policy/eqf_en.htm (accessed on 2 December 2013).

9. The National Agency for Quality Assessment and Accreditation of Spain. Available online: http://www.aneca.es/eng (accessed on 2 December 2013).

10. Hellenic Quality Assurance Agency for Higher Education (HQAA). Available online: http://www.hqaa.gr/ (accessed on 2 December 2013).

11. Estonian Higher Education Quality Agency. Available online: http://www.ekka.archimedes.ee/ (accessed on 2 December 2013).

12. Finnish Higher Education Evaluation System. Available online: http://www.finheec.fi/ (accessed on 2 December 2013).

13. Slovenian Quality Assurance Agency for Higher Education. Available online: http://www.nakvis.si/indexang.html (accessed on 2 December 2013).

14. Polish Accreditation Committee. Available online: http://www.pka.edu.pl/www_en/ (accessed on 2 December 2013).

15. Romanian Agency for Quality Assurance in Higher Education. Available online: http://www.aracis.ro (accessed on 2 December 2013).

16. French Evaluation Agency for Research and Higher Education (AERES). Available online: http://www.aeres-evaluation.fr/ (accessed on 2 December 2013).

17. Quality Assurance Agency for Higher Education. Available online: http://www.qaa.ac.uk/ (accessed on 2 December 2013).

18. Scotland has an independent quality agency. Available online: http://www.qaa.ac.uk/Scotland/ (accessed on 2 December 2013).

19. The General Pharmaceutical Council Operates the Pharmacy Quality Assurance System and This Is a GB Regulator—England, Scotland and Wales. Available online: http:www.pharmacyregulation.org (accessed on 2 December 2013).

20. Northern Ireland has a separate pharmacy regulator—the Pharmaceutical Society of Northern Ireland. This also operates a pharmacy degree Quality Assurance System using the same methodology as the General Pharmaceutical Council. Available online: http://www.psni.org.uk/ (accessed on 2 December 2013).

21. Competency Development and Evaluation Group (CoDEG). Available online: http://www.codeg.org/ (accessed on 2 December 2013).

22. Pharmacy Education and Training in Europe: PHARMINE. 142078-LLP-1-2008-BE-ERASMUS-ECDSP. Available online: http://www.pharmine.org/ (accessed on 2 December 2013).

23. PHAR-QA "Quality Assurance in European Pharmacy Education and Training". 527194-LLP-1-2012-1-BE-ERASMUS-EMCR. Available online: http://www.pharmine.org/PHAR-QA/ (accessed on 2 December 2013).

24. The "Medical Education in Europe—MEDINE" Group Developed Competences for Medical Doctors in a Fashion Similar to That of PHAR-QA. Available online: http://medine2.com/ (accessed on 2 December 2013).

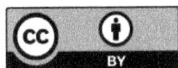

pharmacy

MDPI

Project Report

A Description of the European Pharmacy Education and Training Quality Assurance Project

Jeffrey Atkinson [1,*], Bart Rombaut [2], Antonio Sánchez Pozo [3], Dimitrios Rekkas [4], Peep Veski [5], Jouni Hirvonen [6], Borut Bozic [7], Agnieska Skowron [8] and Constantin Mircioiu [9]

[1] Pharmacology Department, Lorraine University, Pharmacolor Consultants Nancy, 12 rue de Versigny, Villers 54600, France

[2] European Association of Faculties of Pharmacy (EAFP), Vrije Universiteit Brussel (VUB), Laarbeeklaan 103, Brussels 1090, Belgium; brombaut@vub.ac.be

[3] Faculty of Pharmacy, University of Granada (UG), Campus Universitario de la Cartuja s/n, Granada 18701, Spain; sanchezpster@gmail.com

[4] School of Pharmacy, National and Kapodistrian University Athens, (UoA), Panepistimiou 30, Athens 10679, Greece; rekkas@pharm.uoa.gr

[5] Pharmacy Faculty, University of Tartu (UT), Nooruse 1, Tartu 50411, Estonia; peep.veski@ut.ee

[6] Pharmacy Faculty, University of Helsinki (UH), Yliopistonkatu 4, P.O. Box 33-4, Helsinki 00014, Finland; jouni.hirvonen@helsinki.fi

[7] Faculty of Pharmacy, University of Ljubjana (ULFFA), Askerceva cesta 7, Ljubljana 1000, Slovenia; Borut.Bozic@ffa.uni-lj.si

[8] Pharmacy Faculty, Jagiellonian University (JUMC), UL. Golebia 24, Krakow 31-007, Poland; askowron@cm-uj.krakow.pl

[9] Pharmacy Faculty, University of Medicine and Pharmacy "Carol Davila" Bucharest (UMFCD-B), Dionisie Lupu 37, Bucharest 020021, Romania; constantin.mircioiu@yahoo.com

* Author to whom correspondence should be addressed; jeffrey.atkinson@univ-lorraine.fr; Tel./Fax: +33-383-27-37-03.

Received: 30 March 2013; in revised form: 23 April 2013; Accepted: 13 May 2013; Published: 29 May 2013

Abstract: The European Union directive on sectoral professions emphasizes the fact that pharmacists working in member states should possess the competences required for their professional practice; the directive does not, however, describe such competences in detail. The "Quality Assurance in European Pharmacy Education and Training—PHAR-QA" consortium, funded by the European Union, will define such competences and establish a quality assurance system based on them. This will facilitate the tuning of the pharmacy education and training required to produce competent pharmacists in the different member states. PHAR-QA will (1) establish a network of participating pharmacy departments, (2) survey existing quality assurance systems used, and (3) develop competences through iterative interaction with partners. The European Association of Faculties of Pharmacy will use the harmonized competences produced as a basis for the creation of a quality assurance agency for European pharmacy education and training. PHAR-QA will impact on staff and students of European departments; the final stake-holder will be the European patient who will benefit from better pharmaceutical services and better medications.

Keywords: pharmacy; education; quality assurance; competences

1. The Previous "Pharmacy Education in Europe—PHARMINE" Project

The "Quality Assurance in European Pharmacy Education and Training consortium—PHAR-QA" project is based on the work done by the "Pharmacy Education in Europe—PHARMINE" consortium (2008–2011) [1,2]. The latter consisted of 50 pharmacy departments from member states and other European countries that are members of the European Association of Faculties of Pharmacy [3].

Pharmacy **2013**, *1*, 3–7

In a first phase, the "Pharmacy Education in Europe—PHARMINE" consortium developed a set of competences for pharmacists in collaboration with the Pharmaceutical Group of the European Union that represents community pharmacists [4], and also with the European Association of Hospital Pharmacists representing hospital pharmacists [5], and the European Industrial Pharmacists' Group, representing pharmacists working in industry [6]. The "Pharmacy Education in Europe—PHARMINE" consortium also collaborated with the European Pharmacy Students' Association [7].

In a second phase, working with the American Accreditation Council for Pharmacy Education [8], the consortium looked at existing quality assurance systems for pharmacy education and training in the European Union [9]. A questionnaire based on the quality criteria of the International Pharmaceutical Federation [10] and the international committee of the American Accreditation Council for Pharmacy Education [11] was sent out to European departments. Replies were obtained from 28 countries. Just above half have a working quality assurance system. It is likely that those that do not have a quality assurance system did not respond. This underlines the need for a European quality assurance system. Amongst those who did reply, scores were low concerning matters such as evaluation of achievement of mission and goals suggesting, again that a system based on competences is required.

A third aspect of the project was the development of a database of European contacts in pharmacy education and training.

2. The Present "Quality Assurance in European Pharmacy Education and Training—PHAR-QA Project

PHAR-QA (2012–2015) extends the "Pharmacy Education in Europe—PHARMINE" project; it is also funded by the European Union. PHAR-QA is run by a consortium of universities led by the Pharmacy Faculty of the Vrije Universiteit Brussel and Pharmacolor Consultants, Nancy, France with the participation of:

- University of Granada, Spain
- National and Kapodistrian University of Athens, Greece
- University of Tartu, Estonia
- University of Helsinki, Finland
- University of Ljubljana, Slovenia
- Jagiellonian University of Cracow, Poland
- Medical and Pharmaceutical University Carol Davila of Bucharest, Romania

PHAR-QA will build on the competences for pharmacists developed in the "Pharmacy Education in Europe—PHARMINE" project as well as the questionnaire on quality assurance in pharmacy education that project developed. It will further develop the database of contacts in European pharmacy education.

PHAR-QA works in parallel with other initiatives in healthcare disciplines (Table 1). There is collaboration between PHAR-QA and the "Medical Education in Europe—MEDINE" group who are currently developing the third stage of their project [12]. The two groups representing the dental profession, the Association for Dental Education in Europe [13] and the Council of European Dentists [14], are working on a joint position on competences for dentists. PHAR-QA has contacts with these groups.

Table 1. Production of competence frameworks by parallel initiatives in healthcare disciplines.

Acronym	PHAR-QA	MEDINE	ADEE	CED
Name	Quality Assurance in European Pharmacy Education and Training	Medical education in Europe	Association for Dental Education in Europe	Council of European Dentists
Date of publication of competences	>2013	2008	2009	2009

The PHAR-QA consortium will propose foundation and advanced level competences for pharmacy practice and for specialized activities in hospital, industrial [15] and/or laboratory medicine settings. These will be validated by an iterative Delphi [16] interaction with the pharmacy departments in the PHAR-QA network. PHAR-QA uses the TUNING process, an approach to developing quality first, second and third cycle degree programs taking into account the political objectives of the Bologna group [17].

3. Outcomes of PHAR-QA and Their Impact

The competence framework produced by PHAR-QA will be useful in setting up and/or modifying curricula in European pharmacy departments at a time when new areas such as pharmaceutical care are developing.

Another aspect is that many of the science and biomedical competences—as well as the competences required for generic skills such as management and information technology—are common not only to pharmacy but also to medicine and dentistry. Thus the work of PHAR-QA and its interactions with similar groups in other healthcare professions will be useful in the development of common courses for future healthcare professionals.

The framework will also be of value as a guide when considering experiential learning and continuous professional development—two areas of gathering importance. These two ways of developing competences rely much more on skills acquired during professional practice than on knowledge acquired through academic learning. In such a case, a system defined by competences is more useful than one defined by course content.

In collaboration with TUNING [17], PHAR-QA will look at the compatibility of competences in pharmacy with the bachelor-master degree structure proposed by the Bologna group [18]. The consortium will examine the possibility of employment for a graduate who decides to leave university with foundation level competences only—knowing that qualification of the exercise of pharmacy practice as defined by European Union directives requires a 5-year degree course. The latter will not change when the current directive is amended [19].

4. Conclusions

PHAR-QA will produce a harmonized model for quality assurance in pharmacy education and training that will be exploited through the European Association of Faculties of Pharmacy leading to the creation of a European agency for quality assurance in pharmacy education and training. PHAR-QA will impact on European pharmacy department staff and students; the final stake-holder will be the European patient who will benefit from better pharmaceutical services using better medications.

Acknowledgments: The authors acknowledge the valuable assistance of their co-workers: C. Empsen, Lea Noel (VUB), L.R. Manrique, J.M. Aranda (UG), P. Macheras, S.N. Politis, B. Papathanasiou (UoA), D. Volmer, K. Teder (UT), N. Katajavuori, H. Huhtala (UH), I. M. Rascan, A. Obreza, S. Menard, T. Kadunc (UL-FFA), S. Polak, A. Mendyk, M. Kozlowska (JUMC), D. Lupuleasa, F.S. Radulescu, C. Rais, V. Anuta (UMFCD), A. Marcincal (EAFP). PHAR-QA is funded by the European Union [20]: 527194-LLP-1-2012-1-BE-ERASMUS-EMCR. The authors thank the reviewers for their useful comments.

Conflicts of Interest: The authors declare no conflict of interest.

References and Notes

1. Pharmacy Education in Europe—PHARMINE. Available online: http://www.pharmine.org/ (accessed on 23 April 2013).
2. Atkinson, J.; Rombaut, B. The 2011 PHARMINE report on pharmacy and pharmacy education in the European Union. *Pharm. Pract.* **2011**, *9*, 169–187.
3. European Association of Faculties of Pharmacy. Available online: http://www.eafponline.org/ (accessed on 23 April 2013).

4. Pharmaceutical Group of the European Union. Available online: http://www.pgeu.eu/ (accessed on 23 April 2013).

5. European Association of Hospital Pharmacists. Available online: http://www.eahp.eu/ (accessed on 23 April 2013).

6. European Industrial Pharmacists' Group. Available online: http://www.eipg.eu/ (accessed on 23 April 2013).

7. European Pharmacy Students' Association. Available online: http://www.epsa-online.org/ (accessed on 23 April 2013).

8. American Accreditation Council for Pharmacy Education. Available online: https://www.acpe-accredit.org/ (accessed on 23 April 2013).

9. Guimarães-Morais, J.A.; Cavaco, A.M.; Rombaut, B.; Rouse, M.J.; Atkinson, J. Quality assurance in European pharmacy education and training. *Pharm. Pract.* **2011**, *9*, 195–199.

10. International Pharmaceutical Federation. Available online: http://www.fip.org/www/ (accessed on 23 April 2013).

11. International Quality Criteria for Certification of Professional Degree Programs in Pharmacy. Available online: https://www.acpe-accredit.org/international/certificationqualitycriteria.asp/ (accessed on 23 April 2013).

12. Cumming, A.D.; Ross, M.T. The Tuning Project for medicine: Learning outcomes for undergraduate medical education in Europe. *Med. Teach.* **2007**, *29*, 636–641. [CrossRef]

13. Association for Dental Education in Europe. Available online: http://www.adee.org/ (accessed on 23 April 2013).

14. Council of European Dentists. Available online: http://www.eudental.eu/ (accessed on 23 April 2013).

15. Atkinson, J.; Nicholson, J.; Rombaut, B. Survey of pharmaceutical education in Europe PHARMINE—Report on the integration of the industry component in pharmacy education and training. *Eur. Ind. Pharm.* **2012**, *13*, 17–20.

16. United Nations Industrial Development Association. Available online: http://www.unido.org/.../16959_DelphiMethod.pdf (accessed on 23 April 2013).

17. Tuning Educational Structures in Europe: TUNING. Available online: http://www.unideusto.org/tuningeu/ (accessed on 23 April 2013).

18. The Bologna process. Available online: http://www.ond.vlaanderen.be/hogeronderwijs/bologna/ (accessed on 23 April 2013).

19. Vergnaud, B. Proposal for a Directive of the European Parliament and of the Council Amending Directive 2005/36/EC on the Recognition of Professional Qualifications and Regulation on Administrative Cooperation through the Internal Market Information System. Available online: http://www.europarl.europa.eu/meetdocs/2009_2014/documents/imco/dv/vergnaud_profqual_finalreport_/vergnaud_profqual_finalreport_en.pdf (accessed on 23 April 2013).

20. Education, Audiovisual and Culture Executive Agency. Available online: http://www.eacea.ec.europa.eu/ (accessed on 23 April 2013).

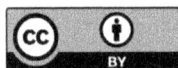

pharmacy

MDPI

Review

The Production of a Framework of Competences for Pharmacy Practice in the European Union

Jeffrey Atkinson [1,*], Bart Rombaut [2,†], Antonio Sánchez Pozo [3], Dimitrios Rekkas [4], Peep Veski [5], Jouni Hirvonen [6], Borut Bozic [7], Agnieska Skowron [8], Constantin Mircioiu [9], Annie Marcincal [10] and Keith Wilson [11]

[1] Pharmacology Department, Lorraine University, Pharmacolor Consultants Nancy (PCN), 12 rue de Versigny, Villers 54600, France

[2] Past-president, European Association of Faculties of Pharmacy (EAFP), Vrije Universiteit Brussel (VUB), Laarbeeklaan 103, Brussels 1090, Belgium

[3] Faculty of Pharmacy, University of Granada (UGR), Campus Universitario de la Cartuja s/n, Granada 18701, Spain; sanchezpster@gmail.com

[4] School of Pharmacy, National and Kapodistrian University Athens, (University of Athens), Panepistimiou 30, Athens 10679, Greece; rekkas@pharm.uoa.gr

[5] Pharmacy Faculty, University of Tartu (UT), Nooruse 1, Tartu 50411, Estonia; peep.veski@ut.ee

[6] Pharmacy Faculty, University of Helsinki (UH), Yliopistonkatu 4, P.O. Box 33-4, Helsinki 00014, Finland; jouni.hirvonen@helsinki.fi

[7] Faculty of Pharmacy, University of Ljubljana, Askerceva cesta 7, Ljubljana 1000, Slovenia; Borut.Bozic@ffa.uni-lj.si

[8] Pharmacy Faculty, Jagiellonian University (University of Cracow), UL, Golebia 24, Krakow 31-007, Poland; askowron@cm-uj.krakow.pl

[9] Pharmacy Faculty, University of Medicine and Pharmacy "Carol Davila" Bucharest (UMFCD-B), Dionisie Lupu 37, Bucharest 020021, Romania; constantin.mircioiu@yahoo.com

[10] Faculty of Pharmacy, Université de Lille 2 (UL), Lille 59000, France; annie.marcincal@pharma.univ-lille2.fr

[11] School of Life and Health Sciences, Aston University (AU), Birmingham, B4 7ET, UK; k.a.wilson@aston.ac.uk

[*] Author to whom correspondence should be addressed; jeffrey.atkinson@univ-lorraine.fr; Tel./Fax: +33-383-27-37-03.

[†] Bart Rombaut passed away in January 2014. This article is dedicated to his memory.

Received: 18 March 2014; in revised form: 22 April 2014; Accepted: 23 April 2014; Published: 9 May 2014

Abstract: The goal of the PHAR-QA (quality assurance in European pharmacy education and training) project is the production of a European framework for a quality assurance system based on competences for pharmacy practice. The PHAR-QA framework will be European, consultative and will encompass the various aspects of pharmacy practice. In this review, we describe the methodology to be used in the project and the first stage in the development of this framework. Using the proposals for competences produced by our previous PHARMINE (Pharmacy education in Europe) project, together with those of other sources, three university professors of pharmacy (Authors 2 through 4) produced a list of three major competency domains that reflect the activities of practitioners: Patient Care Competences, Personal Competences and Management and Organizational Structure Competences. Each domain was subdivided into nine, nine and eight competencies, respectively, for a total of 27 major competencies that were further subdivided into an average of five supporting competences per major competence, giving a total of 140 proposals for competences for pharmacy practice. The 27 and 140 proposals were ranked by an expert panel of seven university professors of pharmacy (Authors 5 through 11). The panel also commented on the proposed competences. On the basis of the ranks and comments, a list of 68 proposals for competences was produced. This list was then examined by the expert panel and a new version based on their comments produced. The latter process was repeated twice based on Delphi methodology. This review presents this process and the 68 proposals. We invite the pharmacy community to participate in the second stage of the elaboration of the PHAR-QA competence framework for pharmacy practice by ranking the proposals and adding comments. It is anticipated that this survey will stimulate a productive discussion on pharmacy education and practice by the various stakeholders (department staff and students, community, hospital and industrial pharmacists, as well as pharmacists working in clinical biology and other branches, together with representatives of chambers and associations).

Keywords: pharmacy; education; quality assurance; competences

---

1. Introduction

The goal of the PHAR-QA (quality assurance in European pharmacy education and training) [1] project is the production of a European framework for a quality assurance system based on competences for pharmacy practice.

The European Higher Education Area (EHEA) was launched in March, 2010. Similar to the Bologna Process (started in 1999), the EHEA is meant to ensure more comparable, compatible and coherent systems of higher education in Europe. The establishment of the European Higher Education Area has led universities to harmonize their educational systems in order to amplify the mutual recognition of degree courses needed for student and professional mobility. This applies to all degree courses, not only pharmacy. Within the European Higher Education Area, the Bologna process developed university programs based on competences [2]. The use of competences eliminates ambiguity and clearly establishes what the student is able to do at the end of the program.

The competence approach is also adopted in European directives. All EU pharmacy degree programs follow the European directive [3] for the recognition of qualifications for sectoral professions. In its latest 2013 version, programs are defined in terms of competences given the evolution in the role of pharmacists towards ensuring safety and efficacy in medicine use, reporting of adverse reactions to pharmaceutical products, personalized patient support and contribution to public health campaigns. Thus, the definition of programs in terms of competences is necessary, not only because of the changes brought about by the Bologna process, but also because of changes in the role of the pharmacist as defined in the EU directive.

The elaboration of a list of competences that are harmonized across different countries, sectoral activities and education systems requires the use of an iterative process, such as the Delphi method [4]. The Delphi method is a process for structuring group communication, allowing a group of individuals, as a whole, to deal with a complex problem. This approach has been used for the elaboration of a framework of competences for medical doctors by the consortium "Medical Education in Europe" (MEDINE) [5]. This EU-funded thematic network used a modified Delphi iterative process to produce a series of outcomes for medical education.

In this paper, we describe the results of the first stage in the production of an EU framework for competences for pharmacy practice using a modified Delphi process. We started with an expert panel consisting of university staff that elaborated through several Delphi rounds the framework to be used as a starting point in the second stage of this process. This second stage will consist in the evaluation of the framework by a much wider expert panel consisting of university staff, students, community pharmacists, hospital pharmacists, industrial pharmacists and others (laboratory medicine/clinical biology, wholesalers, pharmacists working in government and other agencies and representatives from pharmacy chambers and associations).

2. Methods

2.1. Elaboration of the List of Competences

A questionnaire was produced by Authors 2 through 4 incorporating the principles outlined in the 2013 EC directive on sectoral professions. The questionnaire was also based on the framework of competences for pharmacists produced by the PHARMINE (Pharmacy education in Europe) [6] work programme 3 [7] supplemented by frameworks developed for:

- Medical doctors by MEDINE.
- Dentists by ADEE [8]; the Association for Dental Education in Europe (ADEE) was founded in 1975 as an independent European organisation representing academic dentistry and the community of dental educators (from their website).
- Community pharmacists in SW England [9]. The Competency Development and Evaluation Group (CoDEG) is a collaborative network of specialist and academic pharmacists, developers, researchers and practitioners. Its aim is to undertake research and evaluation in order to help develop and support pharmacy practitioners and ensure their fitness to practice at all levels. Among its key outputs are the General Level Framework and the Advanced Level Framework (from their website).

In order to account for future developments in the role of pharmacists, trends in healthcare systems, especially those concerning pharmacy, were also taken into account. We used those outlined in the documents from the European Observatory on Health System and Policies [10].

A questionnaire with 27 major competences was developed as indicated below. The major competences were grouped into 3 major domains representing the main activities of the practitioner.

(I)   Domain "Patient Care Competences", subdivided into 9 major competences:

   (1)   Patient consultation
   (2)   Need for the drug
   (3)   Promote health, engage with the population on health issues and work effectively in a healthcare system
   (4)   Selection of drug
   (5)   Drug specific issues
   (6)   Provision of drug product
   (7)   Medicines information and patient education
   (8)   Monitoring drug therapy
   (9)   Evaluation of outcomes

(II)   Domain "Personal Competences" subdivided into 10 major competences:

   (10)   Organisation
   (11)   Effective communication skills both orally and in writing
   (12)   Teamwork
   (13)   Professionalism
   (14)   Learning and knowledge
   (15)   The global pharmacist
   (16)   Problem-solving knowledge
   (17)   Problem solving; effective use of information and information technology
   (18)   Providing information
   (19)   Follow-up

(III) Management and Organization Competences" subdivided into 8 major competences:

   (20)   Clinical governance
   (21)   Service provision
   (22)   Budget setting and reimbursement
   (23)   Organisation

(24)   Training
(25)   Staff management
(26)   Procurement (medicines purchasing)
(27)   Drug product-process development and manufacture

Each of the 27 major competences was further divided into an average of 5 supporting competences per major competence. Thus, for example, the major competence: "Personal Competences: learning and knowledge" was broken down into 7 proposals:

(1)   Capacity to learn, including continuous professional development;
(2)   Ability to teach others;
(3)   Analysis: ability to apply logic to problem solving, evaluating pros and cons and following up on the solution found;
(4)   Synthesis: capacity to gather relevant knowledge and summarise the key points;
(5)   Capacity to evaluate scientific data in line with current scientific and technological progress;
(6)   Ability to interpret pre-clinical and clinical evidence-based medical science and apply the knowledge to pharmaceutical practice;
(7)   Skills in scientific and biomedical research.

This gave altogether a total of 140 proposals for competences that the panel had to rank.
Complete details of the 140 proposals are available on the PHAR-QA website.
The panel was asked to rank the 27 major competences and the 140 competences according to the following Likert [11] scheme:

(1)   Not important
(2)   Quite important
(3)   Very important
(4)   Essential

2.2. Statistical Analysis

Statistical analysis was performed using parametric and non-parametric methods with GraphPad© software [12]. We used the following methods:

(1)   Descriptive statistics

    i.   Parametric: means and standard deviations
    ii.   Non-parametric: medians with 25 and 75% percentiles

(2)   Tests of normality of distribution:

    i.   Kolmogorov-Smirnov
    ii.   Skewness
    iii.   Kurtosis

(3)   Comparisons

    i.   Non-parametric

        a.   Kruskal–Wallis
        b.   Wilcoxon signed rank test

3. Results

3.1. Panel Members

We analysed the differences amongst the rankings of panel members (Table 1).

Minima (one) and maxima (four) were the same for all seven members. For 6/7, the median was three; means ranged from 3.0 to 3.6 (Table 1). The Kruskal–Wallis test revealed that the median ranking for expert panel Member 7 was different from the other six, but amongst the other six, there were no significant differences. There was a significant correlation between medians and means (test of slope significantly non-zero at $p < 0.05$). The Kolmogorov–Smirnov (K-S) test showed a significant deviation from the normality of distribution. All distributions showed significant critical values for skewness.

Table 1. Statistical analysis of ranking data of the seven expert panel members.

Panel member	1	2	3	4	5	6	7
25% percentile	2.0	3.0	3.0	3.0	3.0	2.0	4.0
Median	3.0	3.0	3.0	3.0	3.0	3.0	4.0
75% percentile	4.0	4.0	4.0	4.0	4.0	4.0	4.0
Mean	3.0	3.2	3.2	3.1	3.2	3.1	3.6
Standard deviation	0.89	0.77	0.72	0.90	0.72	0.96	0.75
Kolmogorov-Smirnov (K-S) distance	0.21	0.26	0.24	0.26	0.25	0.27	0.45
p value	<0.0001	<0.0001	<0.0001	<0.0001	<0.0001	<0.0001	<0.0001
Passed K-S normality test	No	No	No	No	No	No	No
Skewness	−0.31	−0.62	−0.46	−0.69	−0.71	−0.70	−1.8
Kurtosis	−0.91	−0.47	−0.52	−0.51	0.44	−0.63	2.0

3.2. Major Competences

The rankings of the major competences were analysed (Table 2).

Table 2. Statistical analysis of ranking data of the 27 major competences (ranked by mean). Med, median; SD, standard deviation; CV, coefficient of variation.

Rank	Major competence	Domain-number	Med	Mean	SD	CV%
1	Selection of drug	PCC-1.4	4	3.9	0.095	2
2	Providing information	PC-2.18	4	3.8	0.38	10
4	Problem solving: effective use of information and information technology	PC-2.17	3.4	3.6	0.31	9
5	Need for the drug	PCC-1.2	3.3	3.6	0.43	12
8	Provision of drug product	PCC-1.6	3.5	3.5	0.53	15
3	Drug specific issues	PCC-1.5	3.4	3.5	0.23	6
9	Effective communication skills both orally and in writing	PC-2.11	3.6	3.4	0.67	20
7	Procurement (medicines purchasing)	MOC-3.26	3.3	3.4	0.53	16
6	Medicines information and patient education	PCC-1.7	3.3	3.3	0.37	16
12	Problem-solving knowledge	PC-2.16	3.3	3.3	0.2	6
14	Professionalism	PC-2.13	3.3	3.3	0.13	4
10	Monitoring drug therapy	PCC-1.8	3.1	3.3	0.38	12
11	Follow-up	PC-2.19	3	3.3	0.52	15
13	Training	MOC-3.24	3	3.3	0.57	17
15	Learning and knowledge	PC-3.24	3	3.2	0.39	12
16	Patient consultation	PCC-1.1	3.4	3.1	0.57	18

Pharmacy **2014**, *2*, 161–174

Table 2. *Cont.*

Rank	Major competence	Domain-number	Med	Mean	SD	CV%
17	Promote health, engage with population on health issues and work effectively in a health care system	PCC-1.3	3.1	3.1	0.43	14
18	Drug product-process development and manufacture	MOC-3.27	2.9	2.9	0	0
20	Clinical governance	MOC-3.21	3	2.9	0.41	14
19	Organisation	MOC-3.23	2.8	2.8	0.55	19
21	Teamwork	PC-2.12	2.8	2.8	0.46	16
23	The global pharmacist	PC-2.15	2.8	2.7	0.54	20
24	Staff management	MOC-3.25	2.7	2.7	0.39	15
22	Evaluation of outcomes	PCC-1.9	2.5	2.6	0.38	14
25	Organisation	PC-2.10	2.3	2.3	0.9	13
26	Service provision	MOC-3.21	2.2	2.1	0.72	34
27	Budget setting and reimbursement	MOC-3.22	1.3	1.5	0.51	35

PCC, Patient Care Competences; PC, Personal Competences; MOC, Management and Organization Competences.

There was a significant correlation between medians and means (test of slope significantly non-zero at $p < 0.05$). Coefficients of variation ranged from 0–30%. The K-S test showed that for 5/27 major competences ("selection of drug", "providing information", "drug specific issues", "follow-up", "learning and knowledge"), there were significant deviations from normality; in 5/27 ("providing information", "drug specific issues", "effective communication skills both orally and in writing", "learning and knowledge", "the global pharmacist"), there were significant degrees of skewness.

The Wilcoxon signed rank test showed that all the medians for the major competences (except that for the 27th) were significantly different from a theoretical median ranking of one (= not important).

Of the six high ranking major competences (rank: 1–4, 8 and 9; median > 3.4), three were Patient Care Competences and three Personal Competences. Of the eight lowest ranking major competences (rank: 19, 21–27; median < 2.8), four were Management and Organization Competences, one a Patient Care Competence and one a Personal Competence.

3.3. Ranking Data for All Competences

Table 3 shows part of the statistical analysis of the ranking of the data of the 140 competences: the median rank for the three lowest ranked competences (left) was not different from a theoretical rank of one (= not important); the medians for the 6 highest ranked competences (right) were significantly different from 1. The 3 lowest ranked competences showed a wide range of scores from 1 through 4 and very high coefficients of variability compared to the 6 competences that had the highest ranks. Although the Wilcoxon signed rank test comparison to a theoretical value of one (= not important) (W value) showed that the three lowest ranks had scores that were not significantly different from one, it should be noted that this is primarily due to the discrepancies of the positive ranks as negative ranks (*i.e.*, ranks < 1) were all zero.

Pharmacy **2014**, 2, 161–174

Table 3. Part of the statistical analysis of the ranking of the data of the 140 competences: data (**left**) for three lower ranked competences not different from a theoretical rank of one (= not important) and data (**right**) for six highest ranked competences (mean rank = 3.9) (for complete results for the 140 competences). K-S, Kolmogorov-Smirnov; W value, Wilcoxon signed rank test value.

Rank	Lowest	Lowest	Lowest	Highest	Highest	Highest	Highest	Highest	Highest
Competence	Describes the key drivers for national and local service development	Claims reimbursement appropriately for services provided	Ensures the prescriber's intentions are clear	Ensures appropriate timing of dose	Supplies information on documents	Accesses information from appropriate sources	Demonstrates ability to describe the mechanisms of interactions	Provides information that is appropriate to the recipient's needs	Establishes the priority of information provision when it is needed
Median	2	2	4	4	4	4	4	4	4
Minimum	1	1	1	3	3	3	3	3	3
Maximum	3	4	4	4	4	4	4	4	4
25% percentile	1	1	1	4	4	4	4	4	4
75% percentile	3	2.5	4	4	4	4	4	4	4
Mean	2	2	3	3.9	3.9	3.9	3.9	3.9	3.9
Standard deviation	0.82	1.1	1.4	0.38	0.38	0.38	0.38	0.38	0.38
Coefficient of variation	40.82%	54.77%	47.14%	9.80%	9.80%	9.80%	9.80%	9.80%	9.80%
K-S distance	0.21	0.33	0.33	0.5	0.5	0.5	0.5	0.5	0.5
p value	0.2	0.0359	0.0192	<0.0001	<0.0001	<0.0001	<0.0001	<0.0001	<0.0001
Deviation from normality	Yes	No	No	No	No	No	No	No	No
W value	15	10	15	28	28	28	28	28	28
Sum of + ranks	15	10	15	28	28	28	28	28	28
Sum of − ranks	0	0	0	0	0	0	0	0	0
p value	0.0625	0.125	0.0625	0.0156	0.0156	0.0156	0.0156	0.0156	0.0156
Skewness	0	1.4	−0.99	−2.6	−2.6	−2.6	−2.6	−2.6	−2.6
Kurtosis	−1.2	2.5	−1.2	7	7	7	7	7	7

4. Discussion

In this paper, we have presented the PHAR-QA survey modus operandi and the use of a Delphi method with a small-sized expert panel. Thus, this article is about how to determine competences; further articles will deal with the definitive competence framework.

4.1. Likert Scales

As the PHARMINE and PHAR-QA consortia work in close association with MEDINE, we used the four-point Likert scale used by the MEDINE consortium. During discussion with the MEDINE statisticians, they explained that their reasoning behind the use of a four-point, rather than a five-point scale, was that with a five-point scale, the middle ranking point, three ("moderately important"), can be taken as an "easy, no-choice option" and, so, bias the data in the case of long questionnaires. With the latter, the fatigue of filling in the questionnaire may lead panel members to consistently choose Rank 3 for the sake of facility. The four-point scale makes answers requisite in that the responder is obliged to make a value judgement.

However, during our development of the PHAR-QA questionnaire, the following question was raised several times: how does one accommodate for the fact that an expert panel member may simply not know and/or have no opinion on the ranking. This begs the question as to whether the possibility to express the absence of reply should be incorporated into the ranking scale and how. This could be done with a two-stage post-hoc analysis: (1) binary for "reply/no reply"; then (2) parametric/non-parametric for "analysis of ranking". The solution chosen for the Delphi rounds with the European pharmacy community as the expert panel is the use of a four-point Likert scale plus an additional fifth option "I cannot rank this competence". In future papers, the question of how this response can be analysed will be detailed.

4.2. Statistical Analysis of the Rankings

Examination of the data showed that:

(1) There is a lack of sphericity: the variances of the differences between all possible pairs of rankings are not equal. The difference between Rank 1 (not important) and 2 (quite important) is not the same as between 3 (very important) and 4 (essential).

(2) Data are discrete rather than continuous variables: rankings cannot take on any value between two specified values.

(3) Data are skewed to higher ranking values. They do not follow any pre-specified distribution; some data even show an inverse bell-shaped form. In spite of this, there is a significant correlation between median and mean in several cases. This generally implies the normality of data, but in this case is probably affected by the small number of observations. Finally, it should be noted that there is a wide spread in values for the coefficient of variation.

Although the characteristics above would argue in favour of the use of non-parametric methods, both parametric and non-parametric statistics have been used as follows:

(1) Descriptive statistics: reduce and summarize complex data to a few comprehensible variables without losing any of the original information. In this case, parametric statistics (means and standard deviations, coefficient of variation, *etc.*) are more useful, as they are more precise.

(2) Decisional statistics: reveal the statistical importance of such variables while taking into account errors from known or unknown disturbing influences. In this case, non-parametric tests (Wilcoxon signed rank, Kruskal-Wallis, *etc.*) are more appropriate in the case of non-continuous variables, such as ranks, although parametric tests (analysis of variance, *etc.*) do show a certain robustness [13]. It should be noted that in the Wilcoxon comparison of the ranks observed with a theoretical rank of "1" (= not important), the test is affected by the fact that the sum of negative

ranks = 0. This arises because there are no observed ranks <1. As Likert ranks are integral, a rank <1 would be equal to "0", and this would bring in a binary scale of an "important/not important" nature. This is against the philosophy behind the Likert scale, which is used to create nuance in a questionnaire (not important, quite important, very important, essential) and so goes beyond a binary scale.

Albeit, it should be remembered that no statistical analysis can give a correct answer to a wrong question or if used in unfavourable conditions. In order to be valid, the K-S, skewness and kurtosis tests of normality of distribution require a theoretical number of observations >25–30. With seven panel members, this condition is not met, so the results from the tests applied in such circumstances should be treated with caution. This is shown by the fact that in the analysis of the 27 major competences, in some cases (e.g., for "selection of drug") the data did not pass the Kolmogorov-Smirnov test for normality and, yet, did not show statistical significance in the skewness and kurtosis tests. The opposite was also seen: for example, for "effective communication skills both orally and in writing", the data showed significant skewness and, yet, passed the normality test. The design will be more balanced in the future when the expert panel will consist of several hundred persons. This will allow for a more accurate description of distributions and their deviation (or not) from normality. It will also allow cluster analysis of specific groups.

4.3. The Modified Delphi Process and the Rankings of the Proposals (Figure 1)

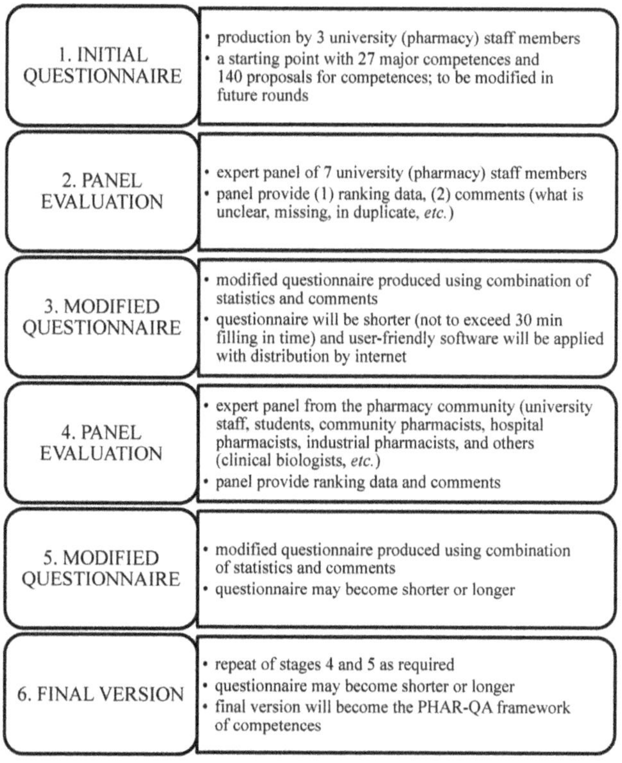

1. INITIAL QUESTIONNAIRE	• production by 3 university (pharmacy) staff members • a starting point with 27 major competences and 140 proposals for competences; to be modified in future rounds
2. PANEL EVALUATION	• expert panel of 7 university (pharmacy) staff members • panel provide (1) ranking data, (2) comments (what is unclear, missing, in duplicate, *etc.*)
3. MODIFIED QUESTIONNAIRE	• modified questionnaire produced using combination of statistics and comments • questionnaire will be shorter (not to exceed 30 min filling in time) and user-friendly software will be applied with distribution by internet
4. PANEL EVALUATION	• expert panel from the pharmacy community (university staff, students, community pharmacists, hospital pharmacists, industrial pharmacists, and others (clinical biologists, *etc.*) • panel provide ranking data and comments
5. MODIFIED QUESTIONNAIRE	• modified questionnaire produced using combination of statistics and comments • questionnaire may become shorter or longer
6. FINAL VERSION	• repeat of stages 4 and 5 as required • questionnaire may become shorter or longer • final version will become the PHAR-QA framework of competences

Figure 1. The modified Delphi process.

The above process has several characteristics:

(1)   It is a two-stage process with the first university staff panel producing a questionnaire that is run through a wider pharmacy community panel at a second stage. This will "even out" discrepancies between the different actors. Thus, for instance, several university staff members gave a low rank to management and organization competences (although there was wide variability on some of these points). It may be that active pharmacists will give such competences a higher rank. The process will ensure that the final framework is universally accepted.

(2)   The initial suggested framework is only a starting point: it may be modified by suggestions to remove or add competences as the process evolves. In the initial stages, it was realised that some competences were duplicates (e.g., major Competences 16 and 17); other competences were not described with sufficient clarity. There have also been changes in the organisation of the questionnaire. At the end of Stage 3 in Figure 1, PHAR-QA will put forward a proposal that represents a consensus (not unanimity) of the opinions of the expert panel members. This constitutes a starting point, and pharmacists around Europe will participate in order to ensure that the final proposed competences will have the widest possible acceptance.

(3)   The final framework will be validated by the large number of responses from pharmacists with widely varying occupations throughout Europe. Thus, the framework will be European, consultative and will encompass pharmacy practice in a wide sense.

(4)   In order to stimulate participation, the time needed to fill in the questionnaire is set at 30 min; thus, the number of questions is limited to 60–70.

4.4. Limitations

The experience of the university staff expert panel outside of academia is unknown. Albeit, in the two-stage process we use, the questionnaire produced by the university staff expert panel is but a consensus starting point for the second stage. It is unknown how far an academically produced starting point questionnaire will influence the final result, *i.e.*, the competence framework produced by the Delphi rounds in the wider EU pharmacy community.

The second stage Delphi rounds will include staff, students, community pharmacists, *etc.*, reflecting the heterogeneity of the EU pharmacy community. The sample of stakeholders should be reflective of the target population. Attention will be paid to collecting a sufficient number of replies from the different stakeholders in different countries in order to allow cluster analysis of possible trends in replies. There is a certain contradiction here with the need to fix numbers in stakeholder categories in terms of factors, such as the population of the country concerned, the relative numbers of staff and students in academia and other factors.

5. Conclusions

PHAR-QA has developed a proposal for a competence framework for pharmacy practice. This represents a consensus (not unanimity) of the opinions of the expert panel members. It constitutes a starting point upon which pharmacists around Europe are invited to comment and validate, giving a final competence framework with the widest possible acceptance.

The questionnaire "The European network evaluation of the PHAR-QA framework of competences for pharmacists" can be found at the website given in [14].

Acknowledgments: PHAR-QA is funded by the European, Education, Audio-visual and Culture Agency (EACEA: [15]); the grant number is 527194-LLP-1-2012-1-BE-ERASMUS-EMCR.

Author Contributions: Bart Rombaut (Vrije Universiteit Brussel) assisted in the design of the project and performance of the research. Jeffrey Atkinson (Pharmacolor Consultants Nancy) helped to design the project and to perform the research, assisted in the data collection, analysis and interpretation, wrote the paper and directed the revision of the paper. Antonio Sanchez-Pozo (University of Granada) helped to design the project and to perform the research and assisted in the data collection and in the revision of the paper. Dimitrios Rekkas (University of Athens) helped to design the project and to perform the research and assisted in the revision of the paper. Peep Veski (University of Tartu) and Jouni Hirvonen helped to design the project and assisted in the revision of the paper. Borut Bozic (University of Ljubljana) helped to design the project and to perform the

Pharmacy **2014**, *2*, 161–174

research and assisted in the revision of the paper. Agnieska Skowron (University of Cracow) helped to perform the research. Constantin Mircioiu (University of Medicine and Pharmacy "Carol Davila" Bucharest) helped to design the project and to perform the research, performed the data analysis and interpretation and assisted in the revision of the paper. Annie Marcincal (University of Lille) helped to perform the research. Keith Wilson (Aston University) helped to design the project and to perform the research and assisted in the data collection and in the revision of the paper.

Conflicts of Interest: The authors declare no conflict of interest.

References

1. PHAR-QA "Quality Assurance in European Pharmacy Education and Training". 527194-LLP-1-2012-1-BE-ERASMUS-EMCR. Available online: http://www.pharmine.org/PHAR-QA/ (accessed on 18 March 2014).
2. Bologna process on the website of the European Universities Association. Available online: http://www.eua.be/eua-work-and-policy-area/building-the-european-higher-education-area/bologna-basics.aspx (accessed on 18 March 2014).
3. EU directive 2013/55/EU on the recognition of professional qualifications. Available online: http://eur-lex.europa.eu/LexUriServ/LexUriServ.do?uri=OJ:L:2005:255:0022:0142:EN:PDF (accessed on 18 March 2014).
4. Hsu, C.C.; Sandford, B.A. The Delphi Technique: Making Sense of Consensus. *Practical Assess. Res. Eval.* 2007, 12. Available online: http://pareonline.net/getvn.asp?v=12&n=10 (accessed on 18 March 2014).
5. Cumming, A.D.; Ross, M.T. The Tuning Project for medicine: Learning outcomes for undergraduate medical education in Europe. *Med. Teach.* **2007**, *29*, 636–641. [CrossRef]
6. PHARMINE "Pharmacy Education and Training in Europe". 142078-LLP-1-2008-1-BE-ERASMUS-ECDSP. Available online: http://www.pharmine.org/ (accessed on 18 March 2014).
7. PHARMINE work programme 3. Available online: http://enzu.pharmine.org/media/filebook/files/PHARMINE%20WP3%20Lisbon%200611.pdf (accessed on 18 March 2014).
8. Association for Dental Education in Europe. Available online: http://www.adee.org/ (accessed on 18 March 2014).
9. CoDEG. The Competency Development and Evaluation Group. Available online: http://www.codeg.org/ (accessed on 18 March 2014).
10. European Observatory on Health System and Policies. Available online: http://www.euro.who.int/en/who-we-are/partners/observatory/eurohealth (accessed on 18 March 2014).
11. Edmondson, D.R. Likert scales. A history. Available online: http://faculty.quinnipiac.edu/charm/CHARM%20proceedings/CHARM%20article%20archive%20pdf%20format/Volume%2012%202005/127%20edmondson.pdf (accessed on 18 March 2014).
12. GraphPad®. Available online: http://www.graphpad.com/ (accessed on 18 March 2014).
13. Raschi, D.; Guiard, V. The robustness of parametric statistical methods. *Psychol. Sci.* **2004**, *46*, 175–208.
14. The survey of the European network evaluation of the PHAR-QA framework of competences for pharmacists. Available online: https://www.surveymonkey.com/s/pharqasurvey1 (accessed on 18 March 2014).
15. European, Education, Audio-visual and Culture Agency (EACEA). Available online: http://eacea.ec.europa.eu/index_en.php (accessed on 18 March 2014).

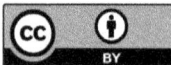

Article

The PHAR-QA Project: Competency Framework for Pharmacy Practice—First Steps, the Results of the European Network Delphi Round 1

Jeffrey Atkinson [1,*], Kristien De Paepe [2], Antonio Sánchez Pozo [3], Dimitrios Rekkas [4], Daisy Volmer [5], Jouni Hirvonen [6], Borut Bozic [7], Agnieska Skowron [8], Constantin Mircioiu [9], Annie Marcincal [10], Andries Koster [11], Keith Wilson [12] and Chris van Schravendijk [13]

[1] Pharmacology Department Lorraine University, Pharmacolor Consultants Nancy, 12 rue de Versigny, Villers 54600, France

[2] Department of Pharmaceutical and Pharmacological Sciences, Research group of In Vitro Toxicology and Dermato-Cosmetology, Vrije Universiteit Brussel, Laarbeeklaan 103, Brussels 1090, Belgium; kdepaepe@vub.ac.be

[3] Faculty of Pharmacy, University of Granada (UGR), Campus Universitario de la Cartuja s/n, Granada 18701, Spain; sanchezpster@gmail.com

[4] School of Pharmacy, National and Kapodistrian University Athens, Panepistimiou 30, Athens 10679, Greece; rekkas@pharm.uoa.gr

[5] Pharmacy Faculty, University of Tartu, Nooruse 1, Tartu 50411, Estonia; daisy.volmer@ut.ee

[6] Pharmacy Faculty, University of Helsinki, Yliopistonkatu 4, P.O. Box 33-4, Helsinki 00014, Finland; jouni.hirvonen@helsinki.fi

[7] Faculty of Pharmacy, University of Ljubljana, Askerceva cesta 7, Ljubljana 1000, Slovenia; Borut.Bozic@ffa.uni-lj.si

[8] Pharmacy Faculty, Jagiellonian University, UL, Golebia 24, Krakow 31-007, Poland; askowron@cm-uj.krakow.pl

[9] Pharmacy Faculty, University of Medicine and Pharmacy "Carol Davila" Bucharest, Dionisie Lupu 37, Bucharest 020021, Romania; constantin.mircioiu@yahoo.com

[10] European Association of Faculties of Pharmacy, Faculty of Pharmacy, Université de Lille 2, Lille 59000, France; annie.marcincal@univ-lille2.fr

[11] European Association of Faculties of Pharmacy, Department Pharmaceutical Sciences, Utrecht University, P.O. Box 80082, 3508 TB Utrecht, The Netherlands; A.S.Koster@uu.nl

[12] School of Life and Health Sciences, Aston University, Birmingham B4 7ET, UK; k.a.wilson@aston.ac.uk

[13] MEDINE2, Vrije Universiteit Brussel, Laarbeeklaan 103, 1090 Brussels, Belgium; chrisvs@vub.ac.be

[*] Author to whom correspondence should be addressed; jeffrey.atkinson@univ-lorraine.fr; Tel./Fax: +33-383-27-37-03.

Academic Editor: Yvonne Perrie

Received: 9 June 2015; Accepted: 10 November 2015; Published: 17 November 2015

Abstract: PHAR-QA, funded by the European Commission, is producing a framework of competences for pharmacy practice. The framework is in line with the EU directive on sectoral professions and takes into account the diversity of the pharmacy profession and the on-going changes in healthcare systems (with an increasingly important role for pharmacists), and in the pharmaceutical industry. PHAR-QA is asking academia, students and practicing pharmacists to rank competences required for practice. The results show that competences in the areas of "drug interactions", "need for drug treatment" and "provision of information and service" were ranked highest whereas those in the areas of "ability to design and conduct research" and "development and production of medicines" were ranked lower. For the latter two categories, industrial pharmacists ranked them higher than did the other five groups.

Keywords: pharmacy; competence; education; practice

Pharmacy **2015**, *3*, 307–329

1. Introduction

Competences, and resulting learning outcomes, are more meaningful indicators than course content or duration. Furthermore, a profession such as pharmacy is defined by competences that are regularly refined in order to fulfill society's demands.

The PHAR-QA project [1] will produce a consensual, harmonized competence framework for pharmacy practice to be used as a base for a QA system for evaluation of university pharmacy education and training at the institutional, national and/or European levels. The framework is in line with the European Union (EU) directive 2013/55/EU on sectoral professions [2] and takes into account the diversity of the pharmacy profession as well as the on-going changes in healthcare systems (with an increasingly important role for pharmacists), and in the pharmaceutical industry. The varying impact of these different factors on pharmacy education in the European setting has been described in detail elsewhere [3–5].

The PHAR-QA consortium is working essentially within the context of 2 of the 5 pillars of the "pillars and foundations of quality" model of the International Pharmaceutical Federation (FIP) [6] namely "context" and "process". Regarding context, the internal environment *i.e.*, the department and university levels, is similar in Europe to that of departments in other regions like the USA, Canada or Australia. The external environment *i.e.*, the political and legal context is somewhat different. Whilst the EU directive 2013/55/EU aims at ensuring competence for pharmacy practice and gives some indications of how education can be organized to provide such competences, it also, importantly, fixes the minimum requirements for pharmacists wishing to work in a different member state country from that in which they received their education and training. This ensures the fundamental principle of the EU that is free movement across borders. EU directives are governed by comitology the process by which a directive acceptable to all members is produced. Within this context, competence frameworks are needed as a tool for international recognition when dealing with the different educational systems and programs in different EU member states. In healthcare more generally, frameworks are designed as educational and developmental tools used both in academia and in practice, both foundation formation and continuous professional development [7–10]. This is the case for competence frameworks that are being developed in individual European countries like Serbia [11], Lithuania [12], Ireland [13], and the UK [14].

The second aspect concerns the pillar "process" which in the FIP document cited above includes nine different activities from strategic planning to appraisal and development of academic staff. This article deals specifically with the seventh of these "process" activities: curricular development and improvement. The framework is intended for a European 5-year pharmacy degree.

Under the auspices of EAFP [15], PHAR-QA brought together several of the major players in pharmacy education from "old" and "new Europe", and from eastern, western, southern and northern Europe (the authors).

The methodology was based similar on that of MEDINE (Medical Education in Europe) [16] in which a framework for medical competences was proposed. Furthermore, PHAR-QA has a representative from MEDINE to help solve the many difficulties of this complex type of project.

In UK English "competence" is defined by the Oxford English Dictionary in four main ways, way 4a being "sufficiency of qualification; capacity to deal adequately with a subject" [17]. In American English, Merriam-Webster's dictionary defines "competence" as "the ability to do something well" [18]. We have used the word in this way with the additional subdivision of propositions for competences into (1) "knowledge" = "being aware of" and thus capable of applying; and (2) "ability" = "capable of doing". Thus, our definition of competence is in line with that of the American Council on Credentialing in Pharmacy [19]: "competence is the ability of a pharmacist based on his knowledge and experience to make the right decision in favor of his patient".

Stakeholders are the major EU pharmacy agencies and associations: PGEU [20], EPSA [21], EAHP [22], and EIPG [23]. PHAR-QA has made contact with pharmacy education QA agencies in

Pharmacy **2015**, *3*, 307–329

the USA (ACPE [24]) and in Australia and New Zealand (PhLOS [25]). This has led to interesting and useful verbal exchange the essence of which has been transcribed into this paper.

2. Methodology

The two main phases of the PHAR-QA project were (1) 3 Delphi rounds within the consortium (authors of this paper), finishing with the development of the PHAR-QA competence framework; and (2) a European-wide survey to refine the framework in a further 2 Delphi rounds and obtain harmonized EU backing for the framework. Thus, the project uses a modified Delphi approach [26]:

(1) Initial questionnaire—round 1 questionnaire was produced by A. Sanchez-Pozo and D. Rekkas using various references [2,27–33] together with comments from the other authors.

(2) Evaluation by the consortial expert panel (the authors)—the round 1 questionnaire was modified in three Delphi rounds, the panel providing rankings and comments on what was unclear, missing, or in duplicate, *etc.*, so producing the fourth version. Nine out of thirteen of the panel (authors) are practicing pharmacists in addition to being academics. Several have more than 20 years of experience as practicing pharmacists. Twelve out of thirteen have a long experience of university teaching of pharmacy, in most cases of 25 years or more. One is an expert in medical education. Once terminology issues were resolved there was widespread consensus on the different visions of pharmacy practice.

(3) The fourth version of the questionnaire consisting of 68 propositions for competences for pharmacy practice in 13 clusters was submitted to a large expert panel (academics, students, and pharmacists from all areas of the profession ($n = 1245$).

(4) The analysis of ranking data and comments on the fourth version, gathered using a *surveymonkey* questionnaire [34], will lead to the production of the fifth version. The ranking data and comments on the fourth version are presented in this article. The *surveymonkey* questionnaire (Figure 1) was available online from 14 February 2014 through 1 November 2015 *i.e.*, 8.5 months. Such a long period was required in order to achieve (a modicum of) balance in the distribution of respondents (by occupation, country, age . . .).

(5) A future second evaluation by the large European wide expert panel will lead to the production of the final QA framework.

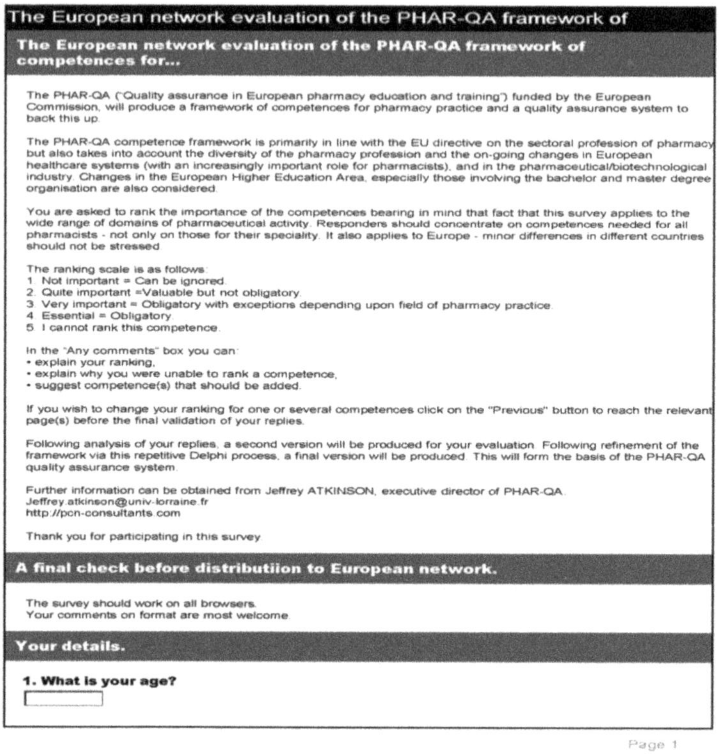

Figure 1. The introductory page of the *surveymonkey* questionnaire.

It should be noted that the first phase of this Delphi process consists in the production of a concerted, harmonious, position paper by a group of experts; this is the essence of the Delphi process [35]. The second phase—the European wide survey—is aimed at producing a harmonized European position on general competence framework.

There were six questions on the profile of the respondent:

(1) Age
(2) Country of residence
(3) Current occupation: community, hospital or industrial pharmacist, pharmacist working on other area, student, academic
(4) If you are a student, what is your year of enrolment?
(5) If you are a professional (licensed practitioner, academic staff...), how long have you been practicing?
(6) Job title

These were followed by 13 clusters in two major domains with a total in all of 68 competences (see Appendix A). Questions in clusters 7 through 11 were concerned with personal competences and in clusters 12 through 19 with patient care competences:

Personal competences

(1) Learning and knowledge.
(2) Values.

Pharmacy **2015**, *3*, 307–329

(3) Communication and organizational skills.
(4) Knowledge of different areas of the science of medicines.
(5) Understanding of industrial pharmacy.

Patient care competences

(6) Patient consultation and assessment.
(7) Need for drug treatment.
(8) Drug interactions.
(9) Provision of drug product.
(10) Patient education.
(11) Provision of information and service.
(12) Monitoring of drug therapy.
(13) Evaluation of outcomes.

Most of those competencies are the same as described in Global Competency Framework, which was published by the FIP [6].

Respondents were asked to rank the proposals for competences with a Likert scale:

(1) Not important = Can be ignored.
(2) Quite important =Valuable but not obligatory.
(3) Very important = Obligatory with exceptions depending upon field of pharmacy practice.
(4) Essential = Obligatory.

The assessment methodology was based on that used by the MEDINE [36]; the even-numbered Likert scale was the same as that used by MEDINE. A pilot MEDINE experiment using a 5-point Likert scale, with a rank 3 = "neutral", showed that respondents tended to "opt out" by replying with rank 3 throughout (M.T. Ross and A. Cummins, MEDINE, personal communication, 2012).

Respondents had the possibility to opt for "I cannot rank this competence" or to leave the answer blank. Finally, they could add their comments.

The distribution of surveymonkey to potential respondents was organized by the PHAR-QA regional directors, *viz* for northern Europe J. Hirvonen, for eastern B. Bozic, for western D. Rekkas, and for southern: A. Sanchez-Pozo. The stakeholders (EPSA, PGEU, EAHP, and EIPG) also distributed the questionnaire to their members. More than one-off emailing was required to obtain some balance in distribution of the profiles of the respondents; numerous telephone contacts and personal contacts were also made. The numbers of respondents snowballed through individual, local contacts.

Results are presented here in the form of scores based on the methodology used in MEDINE: score = (frequency rank 3 + frequency rank 4) as % total.

For example: data for community pharmacists ranking competence number 1:

Rank	Frequency
1	3
2	121
3	480
4	622
Total = 1226	$f\,3+f\,4=1102$ Score = $(1102/1226) \times 100 = 90\%$

Scores give more granularity and a better pictorial representation; they represent "obligatory" rankings. A comparison with medians and means is given in the annex.

Pharmacy **2015**, *3*, 307–329

3. Statistical Analysis

Data presented in this paper are for:

- Overall rankings by six groups of respondents. These are given as means and scores. Although the parametric use of means was probably robust enough under the circumstances, means are given as an indication only and differences were determined using non-parametric methods (see below).
- Comparisons of ranking by community pharmacists with that of the 5 other professional groups of respondents

The differences between rankings of competences or between rankings by different categories of respondents were determined by the chi-square test (confidence level 95%).

Estimated sample size was calculated with a 95% confidence interval and a 10% error [37]. The confidence interval (also called margin of error) is the "plus-or-minus". The confidence level is a measure of confidence. It is expressed as a percentage and represents how often the true percentage of the population who would pick an answer lies within the confidence interval. Most researchers use the 95% confidence level. For example: for community pharmacists (estimated population size: 400,000, 95% confidence interval and 10% confidence interval (margin of error)), the minimal sample size is 97. With a sample of 258 out of 400,000, a confidence level of 95% and a 10% error, for a score of 90% the confidence interval is 4, thus giving a score range of 86%–94%.

4. Results

There were 1613 entries in the *surveymonkey* questionnaire. Of these 1613, 1245 (77%) went beyond the profile description questions (first 6 questions on occupation, *etc.*) and ranked the competence ranking questions (competence clusters 7 through 19).

The numbers of the respondents in the 6 groups are given in Table 1. The relative size of the professional groups was: students > community pharmacists = academics > hospital pharmacists = industrial pharmacists > pharmacists working in other professions. The "other" group included pharmacists working in government agencies (regulatory affairs …), in wholesale, in marketing and sales, *etc.* In all groups sample sizes were well above calculated minimal sampling size (Table 1).

Table 1. Respondents by professional group, and sampling rates.

Professional Groups	Number of Respondents	%	Estimated EUROPEAN POPULATION (× 1000)	Calculated Minimal Sample Size (95% Confidence Level, 10% Error)
Community pharmacists	258	20.7	400 (PGEU)	97
Hospital pharmacists	152	12.2	12 (EAHP)	96
Industrial pharmacists	135	10.8	10 (EIPG)	96
Others	77	6.2	?	?
Breakdown of "others"				
Regulatory affairs, government	27	-	?	?
Consultancy	10	-	?	?
Wholesale, marketing, distribution	10	-	?	?
Lobbyist, NGO	6	-	?	?
Pharmacy chamber, society, association	5	-	?	?
Healthcare insurance agency	1	-	?	?
Not specified	18	-	-	-
Students	382	30.7	200 (PHARMINE)	96
Academics	241	19.4	10 (PHARMINE)	96
Total	1245	100	400 + 12 + 10 + 200 + 10 = 632	97

The ranking of the majority of the 1245 respondents (rank 3 + rank 4: 69.7%, Table 2) showed that the respondents considered the proposed competences were obligatory for pharmacy practice. 12%

considered that competences were not important (rank 1), could not rank or left blanks. 9% either could not rank or left blanks.

Figure 2 shows the ranking of the 68 competences by the 6 groups of respondents. There was overall agreement between groups. Scores greater than 90% were observed for competences in groups 7, 8, 9, 10, 14, 15 and 17, and scores less than 50% for competences in groups 7, 9, 10, 11 and 12. These results indicate that some competences are not considered important although the group in general it is.

Table 2. Global ranking for entire population of respondents, *n* = 1245.

Rank	Number	%
1	2470	2.9
2	14,933	17.6
3	30,132	35.6
4	29,194	34.1
Cannot rank	1764	2.1
Blank	6167	7.3
Theoretical total	= 68 × 1245 = 84,660	100%

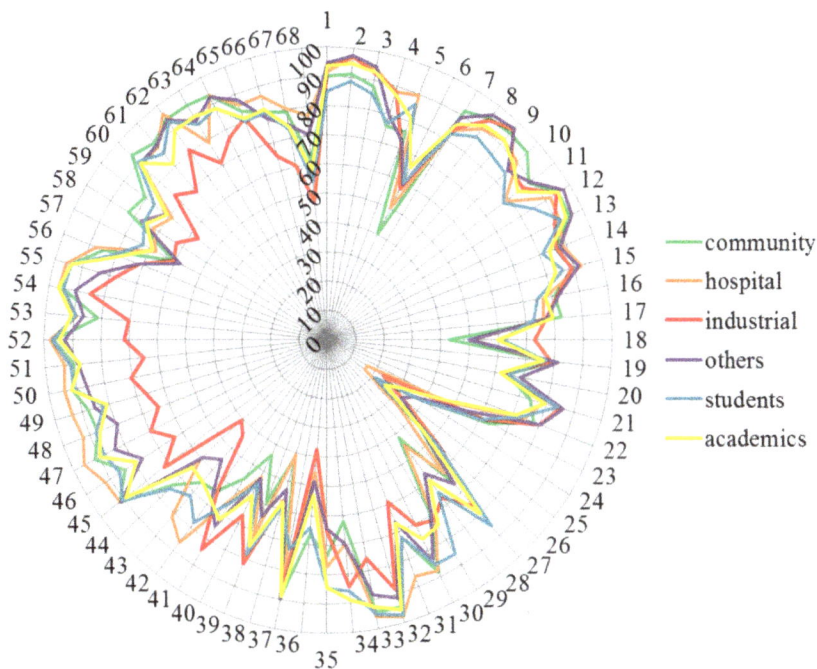

Figure 2. Ranking of the 68 competences by the 6 groups of respondents (community pharmacists: green, industrial pharmacists: red, hospital pharmacists: orange, others: purple, students; blue, academics: yellow). Numbers on the circumference refer to competences (1 through 68). Numbers on the vertical axis refer to % score (0 through 100).

Comparisons between community pharmacists and other groups are given below.

Figure 3 shows that there was little difference in the rankings of hospital and community pharmacists. Ranking for competences 23, 24, 36 and 63 was community > hospital, and for competences 42, 43 and 68 community < hospital.

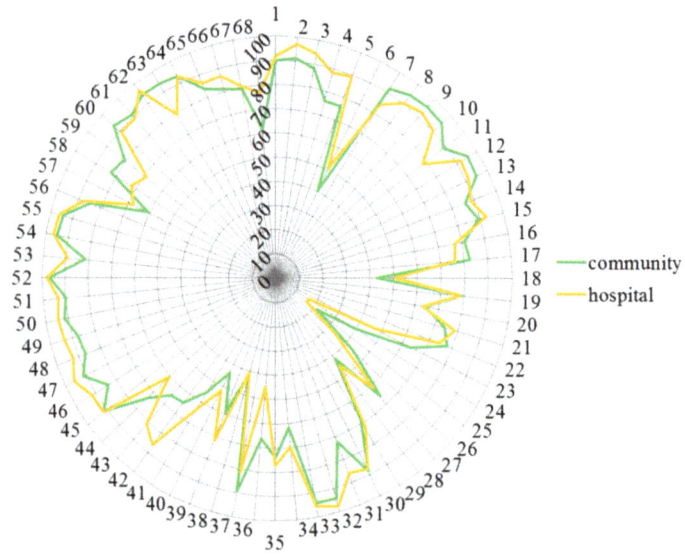

Figure 3. Comparisons of rankings by hospital (orange) and community pharmacists (green). Numbers on the circumference refer to competences (1 through 68). Numbers on the vertical axis refer to % scores (0 through 100).

Figure 4 shows that industrial pharmacists scored differently from community pharmacists. Ranking for competences 24, 30, 33, 36, 43–52, 55, 58, 60, 61, 63, 64, 66 and 67 was community > industrial, and for competences 6, 18, 28, 34 and 38–41 community < industrial.

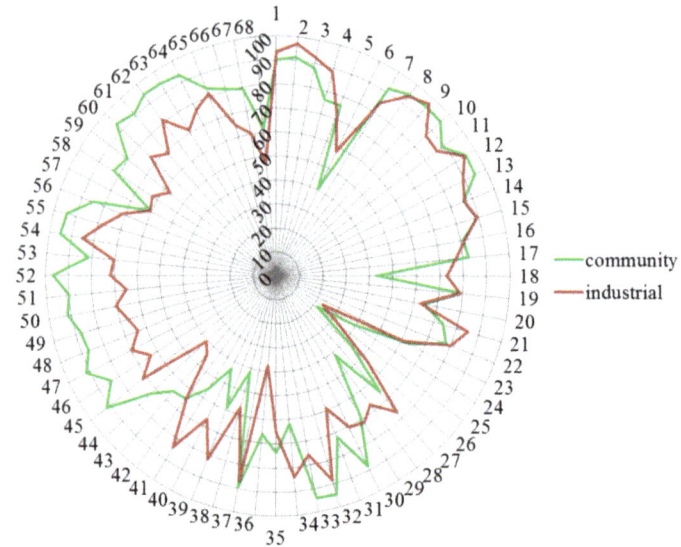

Figure 4. Comparisons of rankings by industrial (red) and community pharmacists (green). Numbers on the circumference refer to competences (1 through 68). Numbers on the vertical axis refer to % score (0 through 100).

Pharmacy **2015**, 3, 307–329

Figure 5 shows that pharmacists working in professions other than community, industrial or hospital pharmacy gave scores similar to those of community pharmacists. Ranking for competence 36 was community > industrial, and for competences 6, 28 and 41 community < industrial.

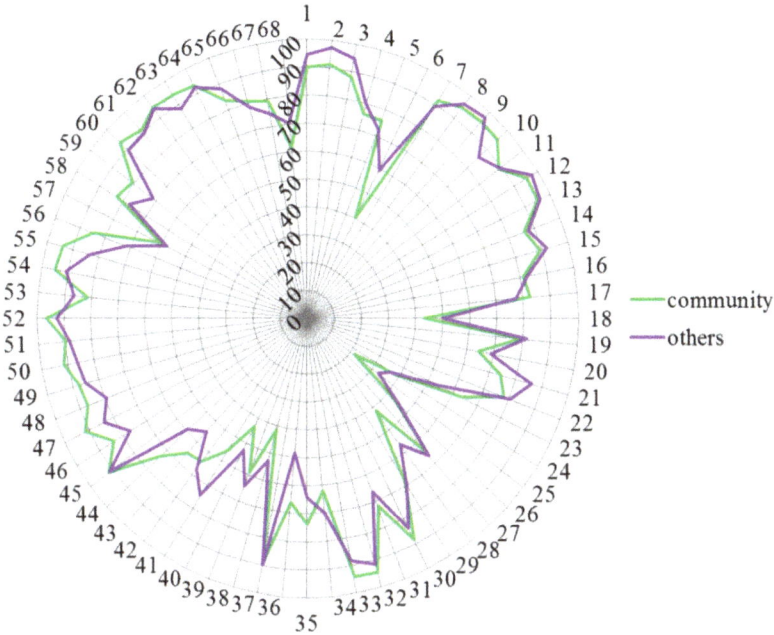

Figure 5. Comparisons of rankings by pharmacists working in other professions (purple) and community pharmacists (green). Numbers on the circumference refer to competences (1 through 68). Numbers on the vertical axis refer to % score (0 through 100).

Figure 6 shows that students often gave higher scores than community pharmacists. Ranking for competence 37 was community > students, and for competences 6, 18, 27–29, 34, 38 and 39 community < students.

Academics often scored higher than community pharmacists. Figure 7 shows that ranking for competence 23 was community > academics, and for competences 6, 18, 28, 34 and 38–41 community < academics.

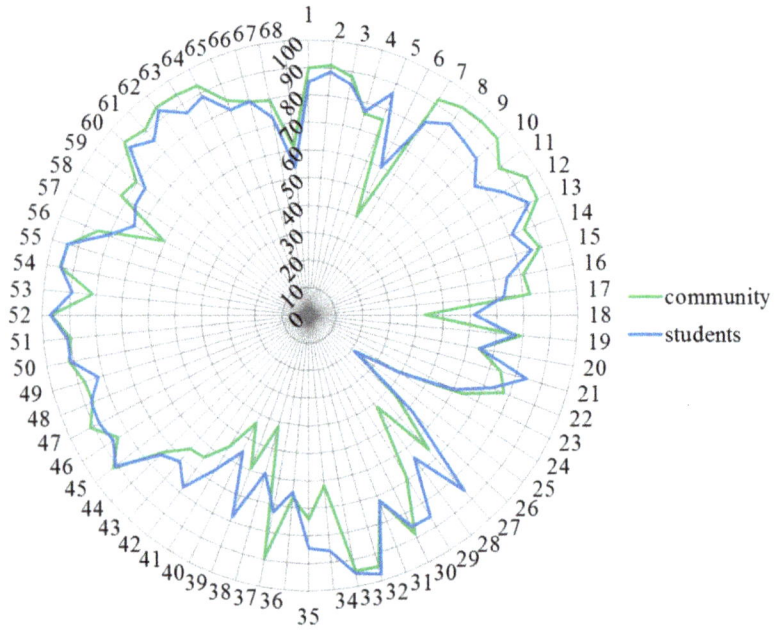

Figure 6. Comparisons of rankings by students (blue) and community pharmacists (green).

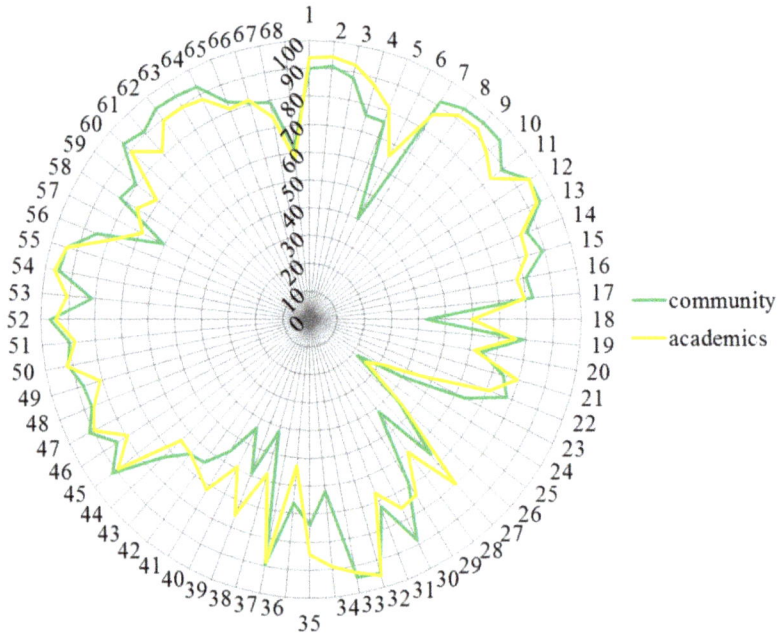

Figure 7. Comparisons of rankings by academics (yellow) and community pharmacists (green). Numbers on the circumference refer to competences (1 through 68). Numbers on the vertical axis refer to % score (0 through 100).

The *surveymonkey* text analysis tool allows the frequency of key words and key terms to be determined thus illustrating the relative importance of the terms. In Figure 8, the font size is proportional to number of citations.

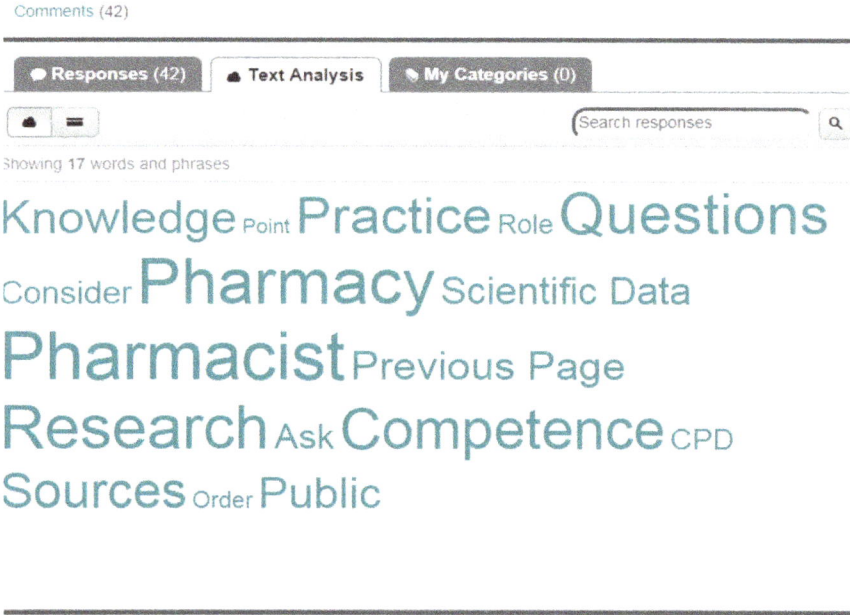

Figure 8. The *surveymonkey* text analysis tool (example for profile question group 10: Personal competences: learning and knowledge).

Comments that occurred frequently included:

- Target audience

  - " ... refer to daily work in a community pharmacy"
  - "focus on practicing pharmacists"
  - "for specialists"
  - "Not really the role of primary care, but important for some knowledge and awareness."
  - "Things that every pharmacist should be familiar with and even more in patient care fields, as in hospital or community pharmacy."
  - "For community pharmacists the above are essential, but for other pharmacists less."
  - "Can imagine it to be important in hospitals..."
  - "For clinical and hospital pharmacists."

- University level

  - "Competences recorded as 'very important' cannot be fully obtained on pre-graduate level and also postgraduate training is needed."
  - "Competence 66 cannot be fully achieved during the pre-graduate training and requires also postgraduate education."

- Difficulties in application

○ "Are subject areas professional competences?"

○ "If not commercially available I would contend that we should change what we are prescribing. I do not believe in 'specials' which in the UK are abused and contribute hugely and inappropriately to our drugs bill."

○ "There are always people who need some special drug which is not commercially available."

○ "Not sure how most pharmacists would be able to manufacture?"

○ "General information on diet or exercise is important but the specific recommendations for the patient should be made by the experts in those areas (e.g. dietician or physiotherapist)."

○ "Information should be basically provided by doctors, before pharmacists."

○ "I am not sure that pharmacists know current clinical guidelines. If medicine is prescribed we give it to patient."

- Suggestions for further inclusions, *etc.*

  ○ "Acquire other competencies for new services like vaccinations in the pharmacy, screening tests (colon cancer, heart disease, COPD, *etc.*) Public Health services in general, NCD (non-communicable diseases)"

  ○ "Services like vaccinations, screenings (colon cancer, kidney, COPD, Heart disease, *etc.*) and others should become essential in the curriculum in order to be able to perform the services in the future."

  ○ "Pharmacist should also provide information about medical devices and other items available in the pharmacy."

  ○ "The knowledge on drug therapies and reactions on failing therapies are core fields for pharmacists."

  ○ "Radio-pharmacy"

- Technical difficulties with the survey

  ○ "In my browser section 6 appears blank"
  ○ "Never ask 2 things in the same question ... "
  ○ "No possibility of open-ended questions ... "

- Language difficulties

  ○ "Too complicated for my simple English ... "
  ○ "I cannot rank this competence for I do not fully understand the meaning of the competence."

5. Discussion

The results show that competences in the areas of "drug interactions", "need for drug treatment" and "provision of information and service" were ranked highest whereas those in the areas of "ability to design and conduct research" and "development and production of medicines" were ranked lower. For the latter two competences one out of six categories—industrial pharmacists—ranked higher than the other 5 groups. The impact of the professional group status on the ranking will be dealt with in a future paper.

The six groups were formed following the end of data collection from respondents. There was no prior separation into sampling groups and no selection. Comments received during European-wide data collection (unpublished) suggested that snowballing was occurring with respondents being recruited by colleagues and friends. Furthermore, the identity of the respondents was unknown; only the computer IP numbers were collected; several respondents could use the same computer.

Thus, the requirement for anonymity in Delphi studies was maintained in the second phase *i.e.*, the European-wide survey. This was not the case in the first phase *i.e.*, the elaboration of the survey by three Delphi rounds within the consortium.

Another question that scored low was that concerned with the subject area "physics". This, however, is not a competence as such. They were included as they are part of the EU directive on the sectoral profession of pharmacy [2]. The question to be asked here was more accurately "adequate knowledge of the following areas (physics ...) in the science of medicines is necessary to support pharmaceutical practice" but once again one is not dealing with competences for practice. Perhaps the best way to consider this is to take the teaching of certain subject areas as an essential, integral part of the acquirement of given competences for practice. This is the position taken by FIP (2012 reference) when they propose that the foundations of quality in pharmacy education are science (or knowledge), practice and ethics. The two aspects "knowledge" and "practice" are well separated and several papers have dealt with the question of how practice relates to knowledge (e.g., Waterfield) and whether pharmacy is a knowledge/science-based profession. The European answer to this question would be "yes" with the proviso that the way in which individual member state countries link practice to knowledge/science is their responsibility and not that of the European Commission.

This freedom of action is also reflected in the issue that organization and management competencies are not included in the framework, nor are time management, financial issues, responsibility for processes and decisions, new tools in the pharmacy profession, such as marketing, category management, procurement, and reimbursement for services. It is judged that such issues are more national than European. Albeit, a question is asked on the "ability to identify the need for new services" with the possibility to develop the answer in the comments box. Several comments were received on future developments in pharmacy practice.

The main difference of the PHAR-QA with the PHARMINE survey is that the former is shorter and more concise. It is intended that the PHAR-QA framework—compared to other national frameworks for example in the UK (CoDEG cited above)—be short and concise and represent a harmonized European version that can be adapted to the national situation in a given member state. The use of the second phase Delphi process ensured that the PHAR-QA framework is consensual and harmonized throughout European countries. This was done by using extensive, random, snowballing recruitment. As stated above, the recruitment was not entirely random as it was distributed by PHAR-QA regional directors and stakeholders—all pharmaceutical in nature—and was thus aimed at a specific population. The survey aimed at balance throughout European countries, professional and age groups. This was largely attained although some groups (e.g., students) and some countries (e.g., Germany) were over-represented in terms of the number of actual respondents compared to the number of potential respondents.

There was a relatively large number of respondents who did not go beyond the profile questions (23%). These were mainly students and this may be related to issues with the English language. The question can be asked as to whether the respondents were suitably armed to reply to the questionnaire. It is unfortunate that 23% of respondents did not go beyond the first six profile questions. However of the 1245 respondents × 68 questions = 84,660 potential replies there were "only" 2.1% "cannot rank" and 7.3% blanks.

The number of respondents (1245) far exceeded the sample size number of 100 respondents estimated for a total population of 632,000 potential respondents. As the numbers in all six categories are large this will allow inter- and intra-group comparisons. In this article, we presented comparisons between ranking by community pharmacists and the ranking by the other 5 professional groups. Many other comparisons are possible such as 1st year students *versus* 5th/6th year students, academics with students, different age groups, *etc.* These will be the subject of further publications. One particular comparison is of great interest: that concerning the ranking in different countries. Ever since the pioneering work of Bourlioux and the founder members of the EAFP [38] there has been a move to harmonization of pharmacy education throughout the EU driven partly by the publication of

EU directives on the sectoral profession of pharmacy [39]. It will be interesting to know whether professionals in different member states have (or have not) similar views on the importance of the different competences for practice.

Regarding statistics, as the ordinal data of the Likert scale has only 4 units (1, 2, 3 or 4), the score was an attempt to introduce more granularity into the results than can be obtained with the use of medians. Scores measure the degree to which competences are considered "obligatory" (ranks 3 and 4). Although this adds granularity it does not convert the ordinal data into ratio data.

The comments from the respondents raised several issues on English phraseology and idiom and these have been corrected in the second version. Words that have a loose definition such as "familiarity" were also removed. Questions that asked 2 separate sub-questions such as "ability to perform and interpret medical laboratory tests" were simplified.

6. Conclusions

The results show that competences in the areas of "drug interactions", "need for drug treatment" and "provision of information and service" were ranked highest whereas those in the areas of "ability to design and conduct research" and "development and production of medicines" were ranked lower.

This PHAR-QA framework does not, however, replace member state law or the EU directive on qualifications for the sectoral profession of pharmacy. The PHAR-QA framework simply represents the consensual opinion of several hundred European pharmacy professionals, academics and students.

7. Perspectives

The project started in October 2012 and will finish in March 2016, thus it is now entering its critical, final stage.

On the basis of the results above PHAR-QA has now produced a fifth version of the competence framework taking into account:

- The ranking of the fourth version of the framework presented in this paper
- The comments of the respondents, namely

  ○ Need for simplified construction of questions
  ○ Attention given to use of easy to understand English

- The question "did we miss anything?" with suggestions for competences to be included (open-ended question)

The revised version of the question is available and readers are invited to respond [40].

The final PHAR-QA framework will be exploited by EAFP that will propose its use in European pharmacy departments and suggest the modalities through which it could be introduced. In a later stage efforts will be made to introduce this competence framework approach to other aspects of education such as continuing professional development and to monitoring of practice.

Acknowledgments: With the support of the Lifelong Learning programme of the European Union: 527194-LLP-1-2012-1-BE-ERASMUS-EMCR.

This project has been funded with support from the European Commission. This publication reflects the views only of the author; the Commission cannot be held responsible for any use which may be made of the information contained therein.

Author Contributions: Jeffrey Atkinson designed, constructed, ran and analysed the survey, and wrote the paper. Kristien De Paepe ran the PHAR-QA consortium. Constantin Mircioiu played a major role in the statistical analyses of the data. Antonio Sánchez Pozo and Dimitrios Rekkas developed the questionnaire. Antonio Sánchez Pozo, Dimitrios Rekkas, Jouni Hirvonen, Borut Bozic, Annie Marcincal and Agnieska Skowron helped with distribution of the survey. Antonio Sánchez Pozo and Borut Bozic provided useful criticism and suggestions during revision of the manuscript. Chris van Schravendijk assured the contacts with MEDINE2.

Conflicts of Interest: The authors declare no conflict of interest.

Pharmacy **2015**, *3*, 307–329

Appendix A

Table A1. Ranking data for 68 competences (*n* = 1245 respondents).

	Number of Competence	Mean Ranking	Median Ranking	Score 3% + 4%
7. Personal competences: learning and knowledge.				
1. Ability to identify learning needs and to learn independently (including continuous professional development (CPD)).	1	3.4	4	89.89
2. Analysis: ability to apply logic to problem solving, evaluating pros and cons and following up on the solution found.	2	3.5	4	92.70
3. Synthesis: capacity to gather and critically appraise relevant knowledge and to summarize the key points.	3	3.4	4	89.70
4. Capacity to evaluate scientific data in line with current scientific and technological knowledge.	4	3.2	3	81.38
5. Ability to interpret preclinical and clinical evidence-based medical science and apply the knowledge to pharmaceutical practice.	5	3.2	3	81.02
6. Ability to design and conduct research using appropriate methodology.	6	2.7	3	55.47
7. Ability to maintain current knowledge of relevant legislation and codes of pharmacy practice.	7	3.3	3	85.96
8. Personal competences: values.				
1. Demonstrate a professional approach to tasks and human relations.	8	3.4	4	91.09
2. Demonstrate the ability to maintain confidentiality.	9	3.5	4	91.74
3. Take full personal responsibility for patient care and other aspects of one's practice.	10	3.4	4	88.43
4. Inspire the confidence of others in one's actions and advice.	11	3.2	3	82.84
5. Demonstrate high ethical standards.	12	3.6	4	91.88
9. Personal competences: communication and organizational skills.				
1. Effective communication skills (both orally and written).	13	3.4	4	92.60
2. Effective use of information technology.	14	3.1	3	84.63
3. Ability to work effectively as part of a team.	15	3.3	3	87.76
4. Ability to identify and implement legal and professional requirements relating to employment (e.g., for pharmacy technicians) and to safety in the workplace.	16	3.1	3	78.43
5. Ability to contribute to the learning and training of staff.	17	3.0	3	77.46
6. Ability to design and manage the development processes in the production of medicines.	18	2.7	3	56.59
7. Ability to identify and manage risk and quality of service issues.	19	3.1	3	77.99
8. Ability to identify the need for new services.	20	2.8	3	64.00
9. Ability to communicate in English and/or locally relevant languages.	21	3.2	3	80.67
10. Ability to evaluate issues related to quality of service.	22	2.9	3	75.07
11. Ability to negotiate, understand a business environment and develop entrepreneurship.	23	2.7	3	56.62
10. Personal competences: knowledge of different areas of the science of medicines.				
1. Plant and animal biology.	24	2.2	2	32.87
2. Physics.	25	2.0	2	23.65
3. General and inorganic chemistry.	26	2.5	2	46.50
4. Organic and medicinal/pharmaceutical chemistry.	27	3.1	3	75.26
5. Analytical chemistry.	28	2.7	3	56.29
6. General and applied biochemistry (medicinal and clinical).	29	3.0	3	75.74
7. Anatomy and physiology; medical terminology.	30	3.2	3	82.86
8. Microbiology.	31	2.9	3	71.21
9. Pharmacology including pharmacokinetics.	32	3.7	4	95.21
10. Pharmacotherapy and pharmaco-epidemiology.	33	3.6	4	91.98

Table A1. *Cont.*

	Number of Competence	Mean Ranking	Median Ranking	Score 3% + 4%
11. Pharmaceutical technology including analyses of medicinal products.	34	3.2	3	78.24
12. Toxicology.	35	3.1	3	77.92
13. Pharmacognosy.	36	2.7	3	56.07
14. Legislation and professional ethics.	37	3.3	3	83.13
11. Personal competences: understanding of industrial pharmacy.				
1. Current knowledge of design, synthesis, isolation, characterization and biological evaluation of active substances.	38	2.6	3	52.39
2. Current knowledge of good manufacturing practice (GMP) and of good laboratory practice (GLP).	39	3.0	3	72.60
3. Current knowledge of European directives on qualified persons (QPs).	40	2.6	3	54.44
4. Current knowledge of drug registration, licensing and marketing.	41	2.9	3	67.36
5. Current knowledge of good clinical practice (GCP).	42	3.0	3	71.96
12. Patient care competences: patient consultation and assessment.				
1. Ability to perform and interpret medical laboratory tests.	43	2.9	3	66.46
2. Ability to perform appropriate diagnostic or physiological tests to inform clinical decision making e.g., measurement of blood pressure.	44	2.8	3	66.27
3. Ability to recognize when referral to another member of the healthcare team is needed because a potential clinical problem is identified (pharmaceutical, medical, psychological or social).	45	3.4	4	88.86
13. Patient care competences: need for drug treatment.				
1. Retrieval and interpretation of relevant information on the patient's clinical background.	46	3.2	3	82.23
2. Retrieval and interpretation of an accurate and comprehensive drug history if and when required.	47	3.4	4	87.83
3. Identification of non-adherence and implementation of appropriate patient intervention.	48	3.3	3	84.80
4. Ability to advise to physicians and—in some cases—prescribe medication.	49	3.2	3	83.10
14. Patient care competences: drug interactions.				
1. Identification, understanding and prioritization of drug-drug interactions at a molecular level (e.g., use of codeine with paracetamol).	50	3.5	4	89.35
2. Identification, understanding, and prioritization of drug-patient interactions, including those that preclude or require the use of a specific drug (e.g., trastuzumab for treatment of breast cancer in women with HER2 overexpression).	51	3.4	4	87.51
3. Identification, understanding, and prioritization of drug-disease interactions (e.g., NSAIDs in heart failure).	52	3.6	4	93.61
15. Patient care competences: provision of drug product.				
1. Familiarity with the bio-pharmaceutical, pharmacodynamic and pharmacokinetic activity of a substance in the body.	53	3.3	3	85.62
2. Supply of appropriate medicines taking into account dose, correct formulation, concentration, administration route and timing.	54	3.6	4	94.03
3. Critical evaluation of the prescription to ensure that it is clinically appropriate and legal.	55	3.5	4	91.87
4. Familiarity with the supply chain of medicines and the ability to ensure timely flow of drug products to the patient.	56	3.1	3	80.26
5. Ability to manufacture medicinal products that are not commercially available.	57	2.9	3	66.57
16. Patient care competences: patient education.				
1. Promotion of public health in collaboration with other actors in the healthcare system.	58	3.1	3	75.53
2. Provision of appropriate lifestyle advice on smoking, obesity, etc.	59	3.0	3	73.07
3. Provision of appropriate advice on resistance to antibiotics and similar public health issues.	60	3.3	3	88.66

Table A1. *Cont.*

	Number of Competence	Mean Ranking	Median Ranking	Score 3% + 4%
17. Patient care competences: provision of information and service.				
1. Ability to use effective consultations to identify the patient's need for information.	61	3.2	3	84.84
2. Provision of accurate and appropriate information on prescription medicines.	62	3.5	4	91.81
3. Provision of informed support for patients in selection and use of non-prescription medicines for minor ailments (e.g., cough remedies...).	63	3.4	4	86.09
18. Patient care competences: monitoring of drug therapy.				
1. Identification and prioritization of problems in the management of medicines in a timely manner and with sufficient efficacy to ensure patient safety.	64	3.3	3	89.01
2. Ability to monitor and report to all concerned in a timely manner, and in accordance with current regulatory guidelines on Good Pharmacovigilance Practices (GVPs), Adverse Drug Events and Reactions (ADEs and ADRs).	65	3.2	3	82.35
3. Undertaking of a critical evaluation of prescribed medicines to confirm that current clinical guidelines are appropriately applied.	66	3.1	3	79.88
19. Patient care competences: evaluation of outcomes.				
1. Assessment of outcomes on the monitoring of patient care and follow-up interventions.	67	3.0	3	74.14
2. Evaluation of cost effectiveness of treatment.	68	2.7	3	59.60

References

1. The PHAR-QA Project: Quality Assurance in European Pharmacy Education and Training. Available online: http://www.phar-qa.eu (accessed on 12 November 2015).

2. The European Commission. The EU Directive 2013/55/EU on the Recognition of Professional Qualifications. Available online: http://eur-lex.europa.eu/LexUriServ/LexUriServ.do?uri=OJ:L:2005:255:0022:0142:EN: PDF (accessed on 18 March 2014).

3. Atkinson, J.; Rombaut, B. The PHARMINE paradigm—matching the supply of pharmacy education and training to demands. *Eur. Ind. Pharm.* **2010**, *6*, 4–7.

4. Atkinson, J.; Rombaut, B. The PHARMINE study on the impact of the European Union directive on sectoral professions and of the Bologna declaration on pharmacy education in Europe. *Pharm. Pract.* **2011**, *9*, 169–187. [CrossRef]

5. Atkinson, J.; Rombaut, B.; Sánchez Pozo, A.; Rekkas, D.; Veski, P.; Hirvonen, J.; Bozic, B.; Skowron, A.; Mircioiu, C.; Marcincal, A.; *et al.* Systems for Quality Assurance in Pharmacy Education and Training in the European Union. *Pharmacy* **2014**, *2*, 17–26. [CrossRef]

6. International Pharmaceutical Federation. FIP Education Initiative. In *Quality Assurance of Pharmacy Education: The FIP Global Framework*, 2nd ed.; 2014; Available online: https://www.fip.org/files/fip/ PharmacyEducation/Quality_Assurance/QA_Framework_2nd_Edition_online_version.pdf (accessed on 12 November 2015).

7. Bruno, A.; Bates, I.; Brock, T.; Anderson, C. Towards a global competency framework. *Am. J. Pharm. Educ.* **2010**, *74*, 56. [CrossRef] [PubMed]

8. Govaerts, M.J. Educational competencies or education for professional competence? *Med. Educ.* **2008**, *42*, 234–236. [CrossRef] [PubMed]

9. Mestrovic, A.; Stanicic, Z.; Ortner-Hadziabdic, M.; Mucalo, I.; Bates, I.; Duggan, C.; Carter, S.; Bruno, A.; Košiček, M. Individualized education and competency development of Croatian community pharmacists using the General Level Framework. *Am. J. Pharm. Educ.* **2012**, *76*, 23. [CrossRef] [PubMed]

10. Dorman, T.; Miller, B.M. Continuing medical education: The link between physician learning and health care outcomes. *Acad. Med.* **2011**, *86*, 1339. [CrossRef] [PubMed]

11. Svetlana1, S.; Ivana, T.; Tatjana, C.; Duskana, K.; Bates, I. Evaluation of Competences at the Community Pharmacy Settings. *Ind. J. Pharm. Edu. Res.* **2014**, *48*, 22–30. [CrossRef]

12. The Association of Lithuanian Serials. Center of Competence of Healthcare and Pharmacy Specialists. Available online: http://serials.lt/news/ (accessed on 12 November 2015).

13. The Pharmaceutical Society of Ireland. Core Competency Framework. Available online: http://www.thepsi.ie/gns/pharmacy-practice/core-competency-framework.aspx (accessed on 12 November 2015).

14. The Competency Development and Evaluation Group (CoDEG). The CoDEG General Level Framework (GLF). Available online: http://www.codeg.org/frameworks/general-level-practice/ (accessed on 12 November 2015).

15. European Association of Faculties of Pharmacy (EAFP). Available online: http://www.eafponline.eu/ (accessed on 12 November 2015).

16. The TUNING Network. Competences: Medical Doctors. Available online: http://www.unideusto.org/tuningeu/subject-areas/medicine.html (accessed on 12 November 2015).

17. Oxford English Dictionary. Definition of "Competence". Available online: http://www.oed.com/view/Entry/37567?redirectedFrom=competence#eid (accessed on 12 November 2015).

18. Merriam-Webster's Dictionary. Definition of "Competence". Available online: http://www.merriam-webster.com/dictionary/competence (accessed on 12 November 2015).

19. The Council on Credentialing in Pharmacy. Credentialing in Pharmacy. *Am. J. Health Syst. Pharm.* **2001**, *58*, 69–76.

20. PGEU—Pharmaceutical Group of the European Union. Available online: http://www.pgeu.eu/ (accessed on 12 November 2015).

21. EPSA—European Pharmaceutical Students Association online. Available online: http://www.epsa-online.org/ (accessed on 12 November 2015).

22. EAHP—European Association of Hospital Pharmacists. Available online: http://www.eahp.eu/ (accessed on 12 November 2015).

23. EIPG—European Industrial Pharmacists Group. Available online: http://www.eipg.eu/ (accessed on 12 November 2015).

24. ACPE—Accreditation Council for Pharmacy Education. Available online: https://www.acpe-accredit.org/ (accessed on 12 November 2015).

25. Stupans, I.; McAllister, S.; Clifford, R.; Hughes, J.; Krass, I.; March, G.; Owen, S.; Woulfe, J. Nationwide collaborative development of learning outcomes and exemplar standards for Australian pharmacy programmes. *Int. J. Pharm. Pract.* **2014**. Available online: http://onlinelibrary.wiley.com/doi/10.1111/ijpp.12163/pdf (accessed on 12 November 2015).

26. Hsu, C.C.; Sandford, B.A. The Delphi Technique: Making Sense of Consensus. *Pract. Assess. Res. Eval.* **2007**, *12*, 1–8.

27. A Competency Framework for Pharmacy Practitioners General Level (CoDEG): General Level Framework, September, 2010. Available online: http://www.codeg.org/frameworks/general-level-practice/ (accessed on 12 November 2015).

28. World Federation for Medical Education (WFME) Global Standards for Quality Improvement in Basic Medical Education BME in English. Available online: http://wfme.org/standards/bme (accessed on 12 November 2015).

29. PHARMINE WP3 Final Report Identifying and Defining Competences for Pharmacists. Available online: http://www.pharmine.org/wp-content/uploads/2014/05/PHARMINE-WP3-Final-ReportDEF_LO.pdf (accessed on 12 November 2015).

30. Medical Education in Europe (MEDINE). Available online: http://medine2.com/archive/medine1/ (accessed on 12 November 2015).

31. International Medical School IMS2020 Report 2011. Available online: http://www.ims-2020.eu/ (accessed on 12 November 2015).

32. Association for Dental Education in Europe ADEE 2009. Available online: http://www.adee.org/ (accessed on 12 November 2015).

33. Eurohealth 2012 Volume 18/2. Available online: http://www.euro.who.int/en/about-us/partners/observatory/publications/eurohealth/gender-and-health (accessed on 12 November 2015).

34. SurveyMonkey (Online Survey Development Cloud). Available online: https://www.surveymonkey.com/ (accessed on 12 November 2015).

35. Goodman, C. The Delphi technique: A critique. *J. Adv. Nurs.* **1987**, *12*, 729–734. [CrossRef] [PubMed]

Pharmacy **2015**, *3*, 307–329

36. Marz, R.; Dekker, F.W.; van Schravendijk, C.; O'Flynn, S.; Ross, M.T. Tuning research competences for Bologna three cycles in medicine: Report of a MEDINE2 European consensus survey. *Perp. Med. Educ.* **2013**, *2*, 181–195. [CrossRef] [PubMed]

37. Survey Software—The Survey System. Available online: http://www.surveysystem.com/sscalc.htm (accessed on 12 November 2015).

38. Bourlioux, P. Erasmus subject evaluations. Studies in pharmacy in Europe. Available online: http://www.phar-qa.eu/wp-content/uploads/2015/04/P_Bourlioux_Erasmus-subject-evaluations-1995.pdf (accessed on 12 November 2015).

39. EUA Briefing Note on Directive 2013/55/EU, Containing the Amendments to Directive 2005/36/EC on the Recognition of Professional Qualifications. Available online: http://www.eua.be/Libraries/Higher_Education/EUA_briefing_note_on_amended_Directive_January_2014.sflb.ashx (accessed on 12 November 2015).

40. The consortium evaluation of the PHAR-QA framework of competences for pharmacists—revised version. Available online: https://www.surveymonkey.com/r/pharqa2 (accessed on 12 November 2015).

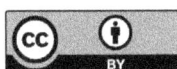

pharmacy

Article

The Second Round of the PHAR-QA Survey of Competences for Pharmacy Practice

Jeffrey Atkinson [1,2,*], Kristien De Paepe [3], Antonio Sánchez Pozo [4], Dimitrios Rekkas [5], Daisy Volmer [6], Jouni Hirvonen [7], Borut Bozic [8], Agnieska Skowron [9], Constantin Mircioiu [10], Annie Marcincal [11], Andries Koster [12], Keith Wilson [13] and Chris van Schravendijk [14]

[1]   Pharmacology Department, Lorraine University, 5 Rue Albert Lebrun, Nancy 54000, France
[2]   Pharmacology Consultants Nancy, 12 rue de Versigny, Villers 54600, France
[3]   Department of Pharmaceutical and Pharmacological Sciences, Vrije Universiteit Brussel, Laarbeeklaan 103, Brussels 1090, Belgium; kdepaepe@vub.ac.be
[4]   Faculty of Pharmacy, University of Granada, Campus Universitario de la Cartuja s/n, Granada 18701, Spain; sanchezp@ugr.es
[5]   School of Pharmacy, National and Kapodistrian University Athens, Panepistimiou 30, Athens 10679, Greece; rekkas@pharm.uoa.gr
[6]   Institute of Pharmacy, Faculty of Medicine, University of Tartu, Nooruse 1, Tartu 50411, Estonia; daisy.volmer@ut.ee
[7]   Pharmacy Faculty, University of Helsinki, Yliopistonkatu 4, P.O. Box 33-4, Helsinki 00014, Finland; jouni.hirvonen@helsinki.fi
[8]   Faculty of Pharmacy, University of Ljubljana, Askerceva Cesta 7, Ljubljana 1000, Slovenia; Borut.Bozic@ffa.uni-lj.si
[9]   Pharmacy Faculty, Jagiellonian University, Golebia 24, Krakow 31-007, Poland; askowron@cm-uj.krakow.pl
[10] Pharmacy Faculty, University of Medicine and Pharmacy "Carol Davila" Bucharest, Dionisie Lupu 37, Bucharest 020021, Romania; constantin.mircioiu@yahoo.com
[11] Faculty of Pharmacy, European Association of Faculties of Pharmacy, Université de Lille 2, Lille 59000, France; annie.marcincal@pharma.univ-lille2.fr
[12] Department of Pharmaceutical Sciences, European Association of Faculties of Pharmacy, Utrecht University, P.O. Box 80082, Utrecht 3508 TB, The Netherlands; A.S.Koster@uu.nl
[13] School of Life and Health Sciences, Aston University, Birmingham B47ET, UK; k.a.wilson@aston.ac.uk
[14] Medical Faculty, Vrije Universiteit Brussel, Laarbeeklaan 103, Brussels 1090, Belgium; chrisvs@vub.ac.be
*   Correspondence: jeffrey.atkinson@univ-lorraine.fr; Tel./Fax: +33-383-273-703

Academic Editor: Yvonne Perrie
Received: 25 May 2016; Accepted: 12 September 2016; Published: 21 September 2016

Abstract: This paper presents the results of the second European Delphi round on the ranking of competences for pharmacy practice and compares these data to those of the first round already published. A comparison of the numbers of respondents, distribution by age group, country of residence, etc., shows that whilst the student population of respondents changed from Round 1 to 2, the populations of the professional groups (community, hospital and industrial pharmacists, pharmacists in other occupations and academics) were more stable. Results are given for the consensus of ranking and the scores of ranking of 50 competences for pharmacy practice. This two-stage, large-scale Delphi process harmonized and validated the Quality Assurance in European Pharmacy Education and Training (PHAR-QA) framework and ensured the adoption by the pharmacy profession of a framework proposed by the academic pharmacy community. The process of evaluation and validation of ranking of competences by the pharmacy profession is now complete, and the PHAR-QA consortium will now put forward a definitive PHAR-QA framework of competences for pharmacy practice.

Keywords: pharmacy; education; competences; framework; practice

---

Pharmacy **2016**, *4*, 27

1. Introduction

PHAR-QA "Quality Assurance in European Pharmacy Education and Training", funded by the European Commission, is producing a framework of competences for pharmacy practice [1] in line with the EU directive on sectoral professions and taking into account the diversity of the pharmacy profession and the on-going changes in healthcare systems and in the pharmaceutical industry. PHAR-QA asked academia, students and practicing pharmacists to rank competences for practice. The results of the first Delphi [2] round show that competences in the areas of "drug interactions", "need for drug treatment" and "provision of information and service" ranked highest. This paper presents the results of the second PHAR-QA Delphi round in the European pharmacy community. A revised version of the PHAR-QA questionnaire was produced following the analysis of the results of the first round [2]. The expert academic panel (the authors) based their revision of the first European Delphi questionnaire on the ranking of, and comments on, the competences proposed. In most cases, the subject matter of the competences was unaltered in the second round survey compared to that of the first round.

Several problems were encountered in the first round [2], and changes were made in order to make the questionnaire clearer. The major changes in the revised version of the survey questionnaire were:

- Questions were simplified, especially regarding matters of:

  . treating one topic per question;
  . simplifying English expressions.

- The section on the subject areas as given in the directive 2013/55/EU (physics, biology, etc.) [3] was removed as these were not considered as "competences".
- Questions on research and industrial pharmacy were reworked given the level for which the PHAR-QA framework is intended: five-year pharmacy degree, not postgraduate specialisation.
- Emphasis was placed on "being aware of", rather than "capable of doing". We used the terms "knowledge", i.e., "being aware of", and "ability", i.e., "capable of doing".
- The second version of the European Delphi questionnaire included an open-ended question for suggestions on matters not proposed that should be treated and other comments.

As the subject area of each competence was not altered, it is possible to compare the rankings of the second round with those of the first.

The rationality behind the study was double. Firstly, pharmacy departments need tools for implementation, but also for the evaluation of programs, striking a balance between a structural approach (subjects, years, etc.) and a competence approach (expected by patients and/or employers). Secondly, following the enormous development and dispersion of pharmacists' professional activities, a diploma without additional information is not enough. This is not a question for the pharmacy degree alone, but is in line with increased expectations in terms of quality, usefulness and employability of graduates [4]. The rationality behind the use of the Delphi methodology was to determine a reliable group opinion from a group of experts with a measure of their consensus [5].

2. Experimental Section

Short Description of the Experimental Paradigm and Methodology

The methodology/paradigm used in the PHAR-QA project has been described in detail elsewhere [2]. A summary is given in Table 1.

Table 1. Research paradigm used. PHAR-QA, Quality Assurance in European Pharmacy Education and Training.

Step	Phase
1	A competence framework based on PHARMINE [6] and other published frameworks for practice in healthcare was ranked (4-point Likert scale) and refined by 3 rounds of a Delphi process [7], by a small expert panel consisting of the authors of this paper.
2	Following the 3rd Delphi round within the small expert panel above, the competences were ranked in two separate rounds by a large expert panel consisting of six groups, European academics, students and practicing pharmacists (community, hospital, industrial and pharmacists working in other professions), using the PHAR-QA SurveyMonkey® (SurveyMonkey Company, Palo Alto, CA, USA) questionnaire [8]. There were 68 competences proposed in the first round and 50 in the second, the difference being due primarily to the removal of the subject areas. Invitations were sent to the 43 countries of the European Higher Education Area that have university pharmacy departments (thus excluding countries, such as Luxembourg and the Vatican). Data were obtained from 38 countries (thus not including Armenia, Azerbaijan, Georgia, Moldova and Russia). In some figures, not all countries are represented, but data from all countries were included in the statistical analysis.
3	The first 6 questions were on the profile of the respondent (age, occupation, experience).
4	Respondents were then asked to rank clusters of questions on competences numbered 7–17 (numbering following on from the 6th question of the respondent profile). Questions in Clusters 7 through 10 were on personal competences and in Clusters 11–17 on patient care competences.
5	Respondents were asked to rank the proposals for competences on a 4-point Likert scale: (1) Not important = Can be ignored; (2) Quite important = Valuable, but not obligatory; (3) Very important = Obligatory, with exceptions depending on the field of pharmacy practice; (4) Essential = Obligatory. There was also a "cannot rank" possibility and the possibility of leaving an answer blank.
6	Ranking scores were calculated (frequency rank 3 + frequency rank 4) as the % of total frequency; this represents the percentage of respondents that considered a given competence as "obligatory".
	The calculation of scores is based on that used by the MEDINE "Medical Education in Europe" study [9].
7	Leik ordinal consensus [10] was calculated as an indication of the dispersion of the data within a given group. Responses for consensus were arbitrarily classified as: <0.2 poor, 0.21–0.4 fair, 0.41–0.6 moderate, 0.61–0.8 substantial, >0.81 good, as in the MEDINE study [7].
8	For differences amongst groups and amongst competences, the statistical significance of differences was estimated from the chi-square test; a significance level of 5% was chosen. Correlation was estimated from the non-parametric Spearman's "r" coefficient and graphically represented using parametric linear regression.
9	Respondents could also comment on their ranking. An attempt was made to analyse comments using the NVivo10® (QSR International Pty Ltd., Victoria, Australia) [11] and the Leximancer® (Leximancer Pty Ltd., Brisbane, Australia) [12] programs for the analysis of semi-quantitative data. In this study and the previous first round study, the word number of the comments was too small to draw significant conclusions.

Each of the individual 3771 entries into the two rounds of the survey was analysed in detail. Entries from respondents not going beyond the first 6 questions (on the respondent profile) were removed, leaving a total of 2773 complete entries for the two rounds, Round 1, 1245, and Round 2, 1528 complete entries.

Several strategies were used to minimize bias. The small expert panel examined the formulation of questions in order to avoid "leading questions" involving suggestive interrogation evoking a particular answer from a particular group. Other biases could arise in the way in which respondents were approached. This has been described in detail elsewhere [2]. In order to avoid bias from a partial response ratio, we defined representative groups and did not send the questionnaire to general populations. However, this by itself could have introduced a bias. It is possible, for instance, that as we used national student associations to contact students (amongst other means) rather than sending the questionnaire to global listings of students, then we harvested results from students motivated to join a student union. The counter argument here is that such students may well be the ones interested in change and evolution in pharmacy education and training with, for instance, more competency-based education. A more general point here is that there may well be self-selection bias by respondents themselves with selection of those more concerned with the future of pharmacy. This may be desirable if the purpose of the Delphi procedure is to direct future developments rather than to confirm present opinions.

"Double replies" were defined as those of respondents with complete replies to the two surveys, separated in time by at least 9 months, both from the same computer Internet Protocol address (IP address) and having identical replies to the first 6 profile questions (age, profession, etc.) of the questionnaire. It was assumed that if the IP address and the replies to the first 6 questions were identical in the two rounds, then the same person was involved in the two rounds. There was no possibility to validate or invalidate this supposition.

3. Results and Discussion

3.1. Presentation of the Results of the Second Round in the European Pharmacy Community and Comparison with the Results of the First Round

The numbers of respondents in the two rounds are presented in Table 2. Compared to the first round, the percentage of respondents going beyond Question 6 in the second round was lower in all groups excepting that of "pharmacists in other professions", where the response rate was higher in the second round (81% versus 48%).

The number of respondents in all groups and in both rounds was higher than the minimum number required to be surveyed based on the estimated European population of each group [2,13].

The percentage of double replies was generally low. It was highest for industrial (16%) and hospital pharmacists (15%; Table 2). Thus, in these two groups, just under one fifth of replies in the two rounds, in all probability, came from the same person. The percentage of double replies for students was very low (0.6%), showing that two different student populations answered the questionnaires in the two different rounds. This reveals a certain conflict in the student group between two of the principles of the Delphi methodology: iteration and anonymity. Iteration would require that the composition of the expert panel remains the same, i.e., that the same people are surveyed, in the different rounds. However, in order to maintain anonymity, the decision was taken not to collect email addresses in the first round and to resend the survey to the same email addresses in the second round (so ensuring that the same people were contacted). We hoped to overcome the difficulty arising from the conflict of "iteration versus anonymity" by using the same global email listings for the different groups in the two rounds and this with the objective of contacting the same people.

Table 2. The numbers of respondents in the two rounds.

Group	Round 1			Round 2			n of Double Replies **	Double Replies %
	Total Number of Web Entries	February 2014–November 2014 Respondents Going beyond Question 6 *	% Respondents Going beyond Question 6	Total Number of Web Entries	August 2015–February 2016 Respondents Going beyond Question 6 *	% Respondents Going beyond Question 6		
Community pharmacists	285	258	91	264	183	69	16	9
Industrial pharmacists	140	135	97	109	93	85	15	16
Hospital pharmacists	173	152	88	271	188	69	29	15
Pharmacists in other professions	159	77	48	89	72	81	4	5
Students	529	382	72	1250	785	63	5	0.6
Academics	267	241	90	235	207	88	21	10
Total	*1553*	*1245*	*NA*	*2218*	*1528*	*NA*	*NA*	*NA*
Average	*NA*	*NA*	*80*	*NA*	*NA*	*69*	*NA*	*9*

* The first 6 questions were on profile (age, profession, etc.). The first 6 "profile" questions were identical in the 2 rounds of the survey. ** "Double replies" are defined as those of respondents with complete replies to the two surveys, separated in time by at least 9 months, both from the same computer Internet Protocol address (IP address) and having identical replies to the first 6 profile questions (age, profession, etc.) of the questionnaire.

In Figure 1 are shown the distributions of respondents by age in the two rounds.

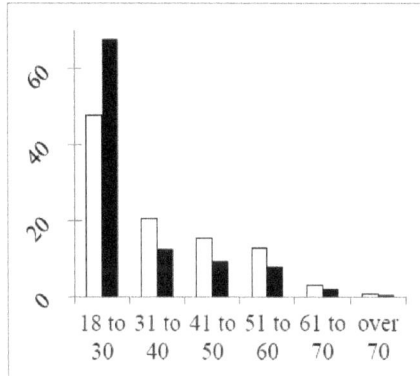

Figure 1. Distributions of respondents by age (%) in the two rounds (Round 1 open columns, Round 2 full columns). The chi-square test of a difference between rounds (df = 5, six groups): 16.8, $p < 0.01$. Chi-square (df = 4; without the student group): 0.6, $p > 0.05$.

In both rounds, 50% or more of the respondents were in the age group 18–30 years old. This reached 68% in the second round due to a much larger percentage of students in this round (Figure 2) and to the difference in the study year of the students between the two rounds (Figure 3).

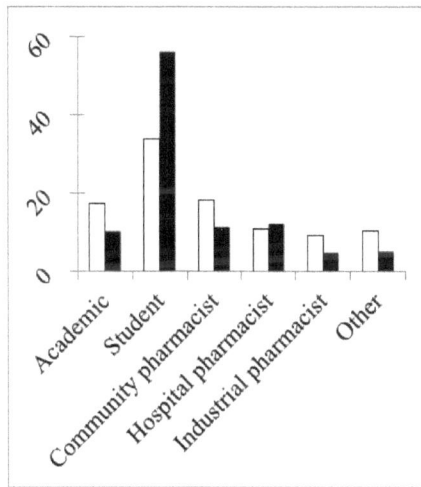

Figure 2. Percentage distribution of different groups in the two rounds ("other": pharmacists working in other professions). The chi-square of a difference between rounds (df = 5, six groups): 13.2, $p < 0.05$. Chi-square (df = 4; without the student group): 2.8, $p > 0.05$.

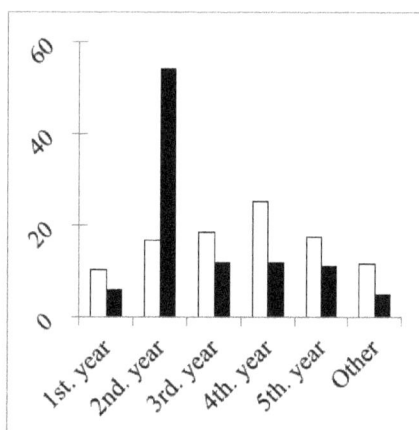

Figure 3. Study years of students (expressed as the % of the total in each round). The chi-square of a difference between rounds (df = 5, six groups): 32.3, $p < 0.001$. Chi-square (df = 4; without the second year group): 0.8, $p > 0.05$.

Figure 3 shows that the main difference in numbers concerned second year students, with almost four-times more students in the second year group in the second round. In other groups the total numbers and the numbers of double replies in the two rounds were similar (Table 2). The greater stability of the groups (excepting students) between the two grounds was illustrated by two other factors. Firstly, the percentage distributions of years of professional experience were similar in the two rounds (Figure 4).

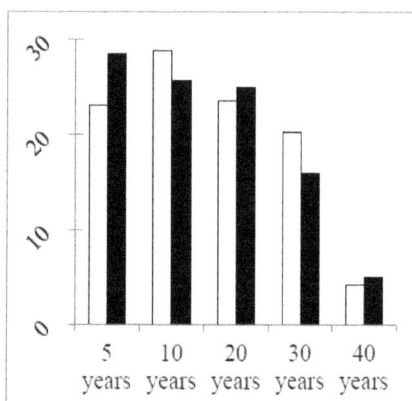

Figure 4. Percentage distributions of the years of professional experience of groups (excepting students). Chi-square (df = 4, five groups): 1.6, $p > 0.05$.

The second factor revealing that the populations of professional groups were similar in the two rounds was the existence of a significant correlation between the numbers of respondents per country in the two rounds in three out of five of the groups: community, hospital and industrial pharmacists (Table 3). Thus, for these three groups, countries returned similar numbers of respondents in the two rounds.

Table 3. Correlation (r) between the numbers of respondents per country in the two rounds. NS: $p > 0.05$.

Group	r	p
Community pharmacists	0.24	$p < 0.05$
Hospital pharmacists	0.68	$p < 0.05$
Industrial pharmacists	0.15	$p < 0.05$
Pharmacists in other professions	0.00002	NS
Academics	0.02	NS
Students	0.0007	NS

The number of students per country in the two rounds determined to a large extent the total number of respondents per country (Figure 5) (data for the top 16 in terms of total respondents/country in Round 2 are given).

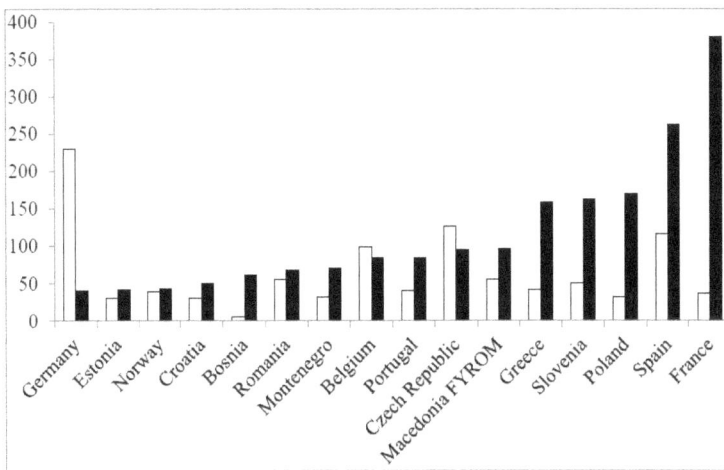

(a)

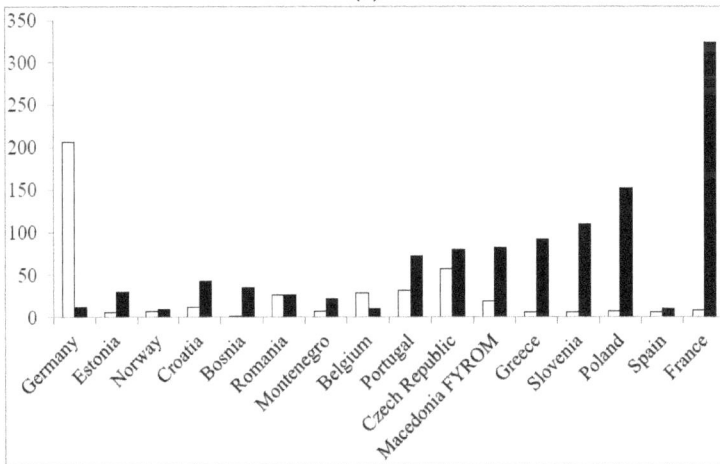

(b)

Figure 5. Total number of respondents per country (**a**); and number of students per country in the two rounds (**b**) (open columns: Round 1; full columns: Round 2).

It can be seen that the large numbers of total respondents in the second round in countries such as France and Poland, for instance, were largely due to the recruitment of large numbers of students in these countries in Round 2. In other countries, e.g., Spain, this was not the case. Thus, although Table 3 reveals that for professional pharmacist groups, the geographical distribution of the respondent population is more or less stable from Round 1 to Round 2, Table 3 and Figure 5 reveal that for other groups, such as students and academics, this is less evident. Two questions have to be answered here: why is there a shift in geographical distribution of respondents in some groups, and does this impact on the global results? The methodology used was the same in both rounds and for all groups. It was essentially based on contacts by email, mainly via professional groups, chambers and associations, backed up by oral contact with individuals and groups. The same email lists were used in the two rounds. Albeit that although the same persons were contacted, the response rate was different, in some groups, from Round 1 to Round 2. Personal contacts suggested that this may have been due to different awareness of the project through national and European publications and to a fall in interest following surveying "fatigue". Although the geographical distribution of respondents changed, this did not appear to modify the correlation between scores for individual competences obtained in the first round and those obtained in the second round (see later). This could be due to the fact that ranking by a given group changes little from one country to another [14].

3.2. Results for the Ranking of Competences and for Consensus in the Second Round

Overall ranking data are given in Table 4.

Table 4. Ranking data for the total population in the second round (n = 1528 respondents).

Ranking	Number of Rankings	%
Essential	25,426	33.3
Very important	27,959	36.6
Quite important	10,708	14.0
Not important	1240	1.6
Cannot rank	1909	2.5
Subtotal	*67,242*	*88.0*
Blanks	9158	12.0
Total	*1528 × 50 = 76,400*	*100.0*

As in the first round, the total for "cannot rank" plus "blanks" was low (14.5%), suggesting that the questionnaire was easy to understand and relevant to practice. The calculated score for the total population (n = 1528 respondents) was high at 81.8%, revealing that globally, 8/10s of respondents ranked the competences as "obligatory". The global Leik consensus was also high at 0.61, revealing that opinions were relatively homogeneous. These values are not significantly different from those of Round 1.

The Leik consensus values for the 50 competences for each of the six groups are given in Figure 6.

Consensus within groups was high (around 0.6) and similar for all groups. Consensus was relatively lower (0.4–0.5) for Competences 20 "knowledge of design, synthesis, isolation, characterisation and biological evaluation of active substances" and 26 "ability to perform appropriate diagnostic tests, e.g., measurement of blood pressure or blood sugar".

Consideration of the Leik consensus values brings us back to the question of bias (which has already been touched upon (see above)). In order to avoid bias in selection, the numbers of respondents were planned to be balanced between countries and professional groups. Since the calculated Leik ordinal consensus between fractions in all groups was high, we considered that this was achieved and that the replies were homogeneous. On a more general basis, in a study such as this, it is unavoidable that certain biases will be present, and this is a possible limitation of the study. The two main elements here are the Delphi approach and the selection of experts. We would argue that the Delphi approach used allowed us to establish an expert group opinion with an acceptable degree of dispersion or consensus. The second element is our definition of experts, i.e., the groups approached for answering the questionnaire. On this point, some may disagree with our choice. Only future studies and data can provide an answer to this question.

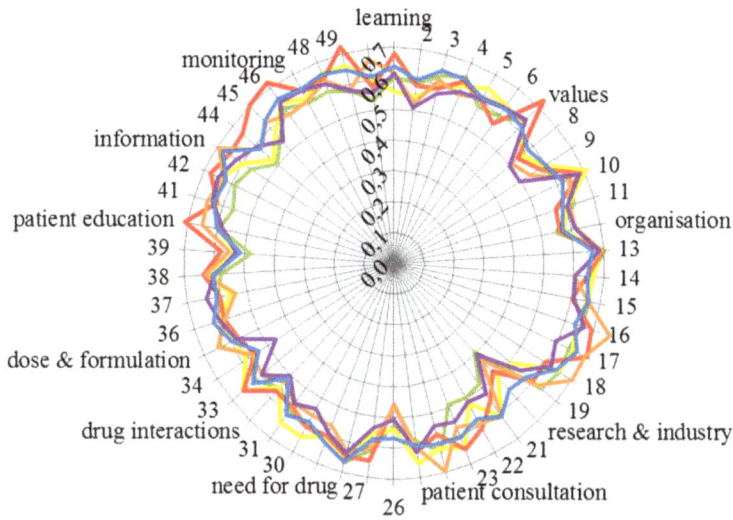

Figure 6. Leik consensus values for the 50 competences of the six groups (vertical scale: Leik consensus, circumference: competence number and cluster; community pharmacists: green; hospital pharmacists: orange; industrial pharmacists: red; pharmacists in other professions: purple; students: blue; academics: yellow). See the Appendix for the details of competences.

The scores for the 50 competences of the six groups are given in Figure 7.

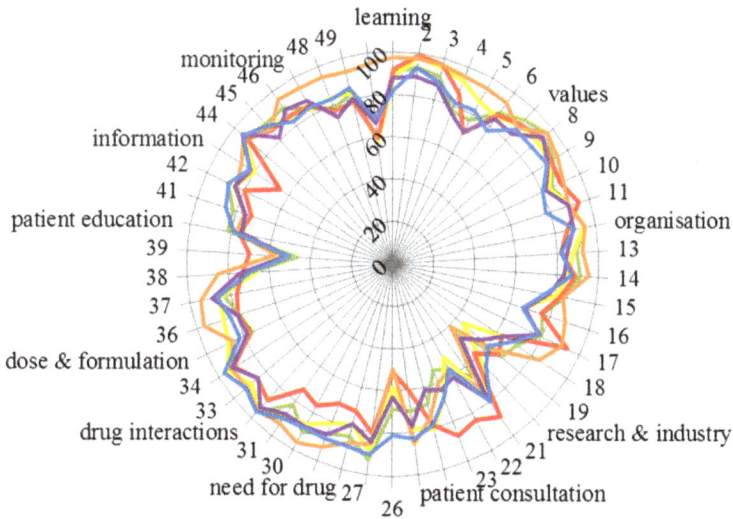

Figure 7. Scores for the 50 competences of the six groups (vertical scale: score, circumference: competence number and cluster; community pharmacists: green; hospital pharmacists: orange; industrial pharmacists: red; pharmacists in other professions: purple; students: blue; academics: yellow). See the Appendix for the details of competences.

Figure 7 emphasises the consensus of scoring amongst groups. Scores were almost exclusively very high (80% or above) except for four competences: 20: "knowledge of design, synthesis, isolation, characterisation and biological evaluation of active substances", 26: "ability to perform appropriate diagnostic tests, e.g., measurement of blood pressure or blood sugar", 39: "ability to manufacture medicinal products that are not commercially available" and 50: "ability to contribute to the cost effectiveness of treatment by collection and analysis of data on medicines' use" (see also the table in the Appendix). It should be noted that there was some disagreement within groups in scoring, as, for instance, Leik consensus on Competences 20 and 26 was low (Figure 6).

Another indicator of global consensus was the Spearman correlation coefficient. When compared with the community pharmacist, groups' score values for the different groups were as follows: hospital pharmacists r = 0.62, industrial pharmacists r = 0.64, pharmacists in other professions r = 0.87, students r = 0.77 and academics r = 0.82 (all $p < 0.001$).

The above correlations are interesting in light of the change in the student contribution from the first to the second round. The proportion of students involved increased very substantially from under 30% (Round 1) to approximately 50% (Round 2). Furthermore, many of those students who responded were only in their second year of pharmacy education. These students may be unqualified to reliably answer such a survey, as they are some distance from actually working as a pharmacist. However the Spearman correlation coefficient for scores for students against scores for community pharmacists is high (0.77) and incidentally higher than that for hospital pharmacists (0.62). Visual inspection of Figure 7 shows that there is a tight relationship between scores for community pharmacists (green line) and students (blue line). Two other points should be considered. In a previous paper on the results from Round 1 [15], students, academics and community pharmacists ranked personal and patient care competences for pharmacy practice. The ranking profiles for all three groups were similar. This was true of the comparison between students and community pharmacists concerning patient care competences, suggesting that students do have a good idea of their future profession. Albeit, a comparison of first and fifth (final) year students did show slightly more awareness of patient care competences in the final year students. On balance, we would suggest that pharmacy students, even those in the early years of study, do have well-founded ideas on the competences required for their future profession. The same paper showed that there were no substantial differences amongst rankings of students from different countries, some with more "medicinal/clinical" courses and others with more "chemical sciences" courses. Secondly, in the PHARMINE study [16], it was found that 9/25 countries provide a substantial part of their training (community and/or hospital pharmacy) in the first two years of study. For example, second year French pharmacy students, who were largely represented in the second round, have a six-week training period.

There were some differences amongst groups, with for instance, hospital pharmacists scoring competence 50 "ability to contribute to the cost effectiveness of treatment by collection and analysis of data on medicines' use" much higher (95%) than the overall average (68%). Another example was industrial pharmacists who score competences in Cluster 10 "research and industrial pharmacy" higher, often substantially, than the global average (see the table in the Appendix).

Given that the subject matter of proposed competences was not substantially altered between rounds, scores for the same competences were compared between Rounds 1 and 2. Linear regression analysis was used (see Figure 8). Two provisos have to be made regarding such use. It is not known whether the variable "score" is normally distributed. Given that the score is a transformed variable calculated on the basis of ranks that are highly skewed to the right suggests that scores may have a non-normal distribution. Furthermore, the exact wording of the individual questions asked differed between the two rounds. In Figure 8 is given as a graphic aid to understanding of the relationships between the two rounds. The non-parametric Spearman correlation coefficient "r" was 0.88, $p < 0.0001$. Global means were 80% for Round 1 and 81% for Round 2.

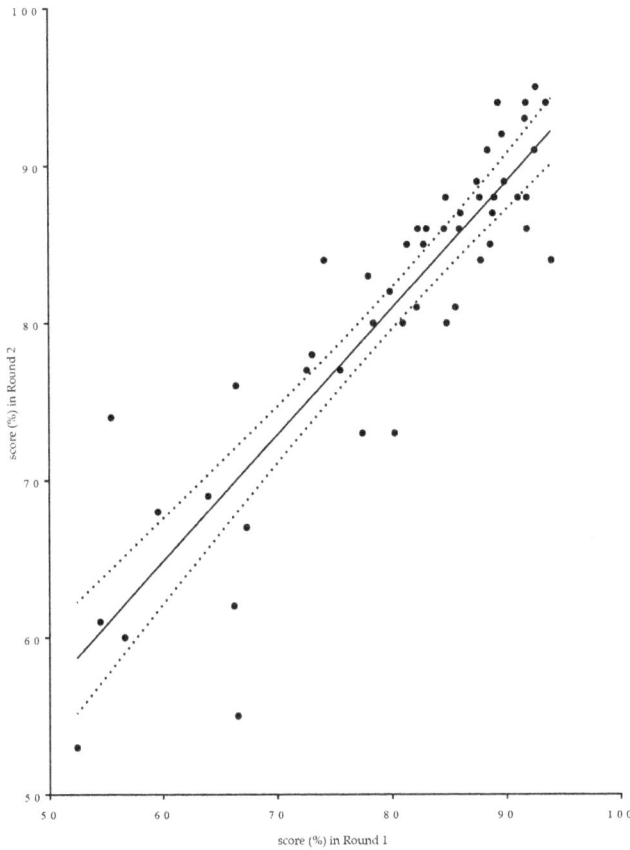

Figure 8. Linear regression graphic representation of the relationship between scores for individual competences obtained in the first round of the PHAR-QA European Delphi survey (*x* axis) and those obtained in the second round (*y* axis) (dotted lines: 95% confidence interval).

In spite of the fact that, in the second round compared to the first, not exactly the same population was questioned and not exactly the same questions were asked, rankings were similar.

The numbers of comments are shown in the Table 5.

Table 5. Numbers of commentators and comments.

Group	Number of Respondents	Number of Commentators	% Respondents Commenting	Number of Comments	Number of Comments/ Commentator
Community pharmacists	183	6	3.3	19	3.17
Hospital pharmacists	188	8	4.3	13	1.63
Industrial pharmacists	93	3	3.2	13	4.33
Pharmacists working in other professions	72	6	8.3	8	1.33
Students	785	16	2.0	33	2.06
Academics	207	11	5.3	27	2.45
Total	*1528*	*50*	*3.3*	*113*	*2.26*

The number of comments was low (3% in the global population), as in the first Delphi study [17]; there were on average two comments per commentator. There were no suggestions as to topics that were not, but should have been, included.

As in Round 1, comments were mainly (31/113) on four topics:

(1) Working environment (six comments). Example: *emphasis should be put on the community pharmacy and hospital pharmacy setting.*

(2) Team work and the definition of the responsibility of the pharmacists within the health team (14 comments). Example: *clearly know what the pharmacist is responsible for.* One community pharmacist suggested that pharmacists were ideally suited to be the "coordinator" of the health team.

(3) Legal and other limits to the pharmacist's responsibility (seven comments). Examples: *diagnosis is the responsibility of doctors; pharmacists in Latvia mostly work in chain-pharmacies . . . where owners and managers have no pharmaceutical education.*

(4) Use of information technology (four comments). Example: *ability to find appropriate sources and use electronic platforms.*

The other 82 comments were on very diverse topics. This prevented the evaluation of any definitive pattern in comments with the use of semi-quantitative data analysis software.

4. Conclusions

The essence of the methodology of the PHAR-QA approach can be summarized as follows. We started with a framework based on PHARMINE [6]. To this, we added elements from frameworks used by other healthcare professions, doctors [9] and dentists [18]. Finally, frameworks used in other countries, such as the U.K. [19], Canada [20] and Australia [21], for pharmacists were used. This was refined by three Delphi rounds within a small expert panel (authors of this paper). This approach has been used in previous studies and can be criticised on the basis that there is no real "transfer" of the framework from academics to practitioners. Such a transfer was attempted in the MEDINE study in which the framework proposed by the academic community passed through a (single) Delphi round within a large expert panel consisting of European medical practitioners and students. In PHAR-QA, such validation was taken further by having two Delphi rounds with a large expert panel of European pharmacy professionals, academics and students. The aim of this two-round approach was to harmonise, as well as validate the competence framework and ensure that a framework elaborated by an academic expert panel would be adopted by the European pharmacy community.

The question can be asked as to whether such a "double Delphi" process works. There are several indications that this is the case. Firstly, the ranks given varied widely from 41%–99%. Respondents did not give a "global" rank that was more or less the same for all competences, and yet, secondly, there was good consensus within the groups and amongst the groups. Thirdly, except for students, there were a significant number of double replies. Fourthly, again, except for students, the profiles of the responding groups in terms of age, country of origin, years of experience, etc., were similar in the two rounds. Thus although, for the sake of anonymity, we did not collect email addresses in the first round and send the second version of the survey to the same email addresses, it would appear that in the professional groups, the profiles of respondents are similar in the two rounds. Fifthly, the replies obtained in the two rounds were highly correlated (see Figure 8).

One proviso on the statistical methodology used has to be added. On several occasions in this study, parametric statistics have been used for variables that may not necessarily follow a normal distribution. This was done in the analysis of the data of the first round [2] and justified on such occasions by the fact that parametric tests are robust [22].

Finally, a few observations on the use of the PHAR-QA competence framework are presented below:

- A good starting point for the adoption of the competence framework is to match existing curriculum of a department to the framework; this approach has previously been used to match outcomes to curricula, and the methodology has been published [23].
- Building a curriculum based on the PHAR-QA competence framework could be guided by the following:

  ○ Core curriculum: the fundamental, bachelor curriculum could be based, amongst others, on the clusters of competences with the highest ranking scores, *viz*, 12: "need for drug treatment", 13: "drug interactions" and 16: "provision of information and service".

  ○ Specialisation in the advanced, master curriculum could include, for instance,

    ▪ for community pharmacists: Competences 32 "ability to identify and prioritise drug-drug interactions and advise appropriate changes to medication" and 34 "ability to identify and prioritise drug-disease interactions (e.g., NSAIDs in heart failure) and advise on appropriate changes to medication"
    ▪ for hospital pharmacists: Competences 36 "ability to recommend interchangeability of drugs based on in-depth understanding and knowledge of bioequivalence, bio-similarity and therapeutic equivalence of drugs" and 50 "ability to contribute to the cost effectiveness of treatment by collection and analysis of data on medicines' use"
    ▪ for industrial pharmacists; Competences 21 "knowledge of good manufacturing practice and of good laboratory practice" and 23 "knowledge of drug registration, licensing and marketing"

  ○ The ways in which the various competences are taught are diverse. For instance, for personal competence Clusters 8 "values" and 9 "communication and organisational skills", the role of the traineeship monitor is uppermost. The way in which this is to be developed needs to be harmonized within the EU, but the finer details would be up to individual faculties.

The overall conclusion of the PHAR-QA study is that pharmacists, regardless of their career path, have a great deal in common; all are seeking for improvements in their services to patients. Their different perspectives in certain areas represent a solid starting point for steering the necessary changes through discussions within their professional organisations and faculties. PHAR-QA intended to bridge the different career paths through consensus; thus, all concerned can view these findings as an opportunity to further strengthen the scientific role of the pharmacist.

Acknowledgments: With the support of the Lifelong Learning programme of the European Union: 527194-LLP-1–2012–1-BE-ERASMUS-EMCR. This project has been funded with support from the European Commission. This publication reflects the views only of the author; the Commission cannot be held responsible for any use that may be made of the information contained therein.

Author Contributions: Jeffrey Atkinson designed, constructed, ran and analysed the survey and wrote the paper. Kristien De Paepe ran the PHAR-QA consortium. Constantin Mircioiu played a major role in the statistical analyses of the data. Antonio Sánchez Pozo and Dimitrios Rekkas developed the questionnaire. Antonio Sánchez Pozo, Dimitrios Rekkas, Jouni Hirvonen, Borut Bozic, Annie Marcincal and Agnieska Skowron helped with the distribution of the survey. All authors provided useful criticism and suggestions during revision of the manuscript. Chris van Schravendijk assured the contacts with MEDINE2.

Conflicts of Interest: The authors declare no conflict of interest.

Appendix

Table A1. Ranking of Competences.

Question	Competence	Community	Industrial	Hospital	Others	Students	Academics	Mean
	7. Personal competences: learning and knowledge.							88
1	1. Ability to identify learning needs and to learn independently (including continuous professional development (CPD)).	90	91	97	87	82	88	89
2	2. Ability to apply logic to problem solving.	93	99	97	89	93	98	95
3	3. Ability to critically appraise relevant knowledge and to summarise the key points.	91	97	97	87	88	95	92
4	4. Ability to evaluate scientific data in line with current scientific and technological knowledge.	78	86	95	76	81	93	85
5	5. Ability to apply preclinical and clinical evidence-based medical science to pharmaceutical practice.	77	70	94	71	82	87	80
6	6. Ability to apply current knowledge of relevant legislation and codes of pharmacy practice.	88	87	94	84	77	85	86
	8. Personal competences: values.							89
7	1. A professional approach to tasks and human relations.	93	90	88	84	87	89	88
8	2. Ability to maintain confidentiality.	96	93	97	94	87	90	93
9	3. Ability to take full responsibility for patient care.	92	90	94	89	88	90	91
10	4. Ability to inspire the confidence of others in one's actions and advice.	85	90	91	82	80	83	85
11	5. Knowledge of appropriate legislation and of ethics.	90	94	90	89	78	90	88
	9. Personal competences: communication and organisational skills.							79
12	1. Ability to communicate effectively, both oral and written, in the locally relevant language.	95	86	94	89	89	94	91
13	2. Ability to effectively use information technology.	89	81	92	84	82	88	86
14	3. Ability to work effectively as part of a team.	91	88	95	83	87	85	88
15	4. Ability to implement general legal requirements that impact upon the practice of pharmacy (e.g., health and safety legislation, employment law).	84	83	84	77	74	80	80
16	5. Ability to contribute to the training of staff.	76	76	88	67	66	67	73
17	6. Ability to manage risk and quality of service issues.	80	93	90	78	78	79	83
18	7. Ability to identify the need for new services.	72	63	84	63	69	63	69
19	8. Ability to understand a business environment and develop entrepreneurship.	69	67	63	56	60	44	60
	10. Personal competences: research and industrial pharmacy.							66
20	1. Knowledge of design, synthesis, isolation, characterisation and biological evaluation of active substances.	44	58	41	48	66	63	53

Table A1. *Cont.*

Question	Competence	Community	Industrial	Hospital	Others	Students	Academics	Mean
21	2. Knowledge of good manufacturing practice and of good laboratory practice.	65	89	73	78	81	76	77
22	3. Knowledge of European directives on qualified persons.	56	84	57	61	57	51	61
23	4. Knowledge of drug registration, licensing and marketing.	54	87	60	64	68	67	67
24	5. Knowledge of the importance of research in pharmaceutical development and practice.	68	78	74	62	78	81	74
	11. Patient care competences: patient consultation and assessment.							75
25	1. Ability to interpret basic medical laboratory tests.	70	60	86	77	83	79	76
26	2. Ability to perform appropriate diagnostic tests, e.g., measurement of blood pressure or blood sugar.	69	51	49	63	81	59	62
27	3. Ability to recognise when referral to another member of the healthcare team is needed.	93	81	86	84	91	90	87
	12. Patient care competences: need for drug treatment.							85
28	1. Ability to retrieve and interpret information on the patient's clinical background.	84	72	87	78	89	78	81
29	2. Ability to compile and interpret a comprehensive drug history for an individual patient.	86	71	93	86	89	81	84
30	3. Ability to identify non-adherence to medicine therapy and make an appropriate intervention.	91	76	96	88	89	87	88
31	4. Ability to advise to physicians on the appropriateness of prescribed medicines and, in some cases, to prescribe medication.	83	74	93	88	90	89	86
	13. Patient care competences: drug interactions.							92
32	1. Ability to identify and prioritise drug-drug interactions and advise appropriate changes to medication.	96	89	95	94	96	94	94
33	2. Ability to identify and prioritise drug-patient interactions, including those that prevent or require the use of a specific drug, based on pharmaco-genetics, and advise on appropriate changes to medication.	90	85	92	85	92	89	89
34	3. Ability to identify and prioritise drug-disease interactions (e.g., NSAIDs in heart failure) and advise on appropriate changes to medication.	96	91	93	92	97	95	94
	14. Patient care competences: drug dose and formulation.							76
35	1. Knowledge of the bio-pharmaceutical, pharmacodynamic and pharmacokinetic activity of a substance in the body.	75	76	86	78	82	88	81
36	2. Ability to recommend interchangeability of drugs based on in-depth understanding and knowledge of bioequivalence, bio-similarity and therapeutic equivalence of drugs.	79	79	96	79	83	86	84
37	3. Ability to undertake a critical evaluation of a prescription ensuring that it is clinically appropriate and legally valid.	83	77	95	89	87	86	86
38	4. Knowledge of the supply chain of medicines thus ensuring timely flow of quality drug products to the patient.	69	73	85	75	69	66	73
39	5. Ability to manufacture medicinal products that are not commercially available.	46	70	57	52	51	57	55
	15. Patient care competences: patient education.							80
40	1. Ability to promote public health in collaboration with other professionals within the healthcare system.	82	76	78	75	79	73	77

Table A1. *Cont.*

Question	Competence	Community	Industrial	Hospital	Others	Students	Academics	Mean
41	2. Ability to provide appropriate lifestyle advice to improve patient outcomes (e.g., advice on smoking, obesity, etc.).	81	72	76	75	85	76	78
42	3. Ability to use pharmaceutical knowledge and provide evidence-based advice on public health issues involving medicines.	89	80	84	85	88	85	85
	16. Patient care competences: provision of information and service.							87
43	1. Ability to use effective consultations to identify the patient's need for information.	82	65	87	82	82	79	80
44	2. Ability to provide accurate and appropriate information on prescription medicines.	93	92	94	95	94	94	94
45	3. Ability to provide evidence-based support for patients in selection and use of non-prescription medicines.	90	86	87	81	88	89	87
	17. Patient care competences: monitoring of drug therapy.							81
46	1. Ability to identify and prioritise problems in the management of medicines in a timely and effective manner and so ensure patient safety.	91	86	95	89	82	85	88
47	2. Ability to monitor and report adverse drug events and adverse drug reactions (ADEs and ADRs) to all concerned, in a timely manner, and in accordance with current regulatory guidelines on good pharmacovigilance practices (GVPs).	83	85	94	87	84	83	86
48	3. Ability to undertake a critical evaluation of prescribed medicines to confirm that current clinical guidelines are appropriately applied.	78	77	94	74	83	83	82
49	4. Ability to monitor patient care outcomes to optimise treatment in collaboration with the prescriber.	83	78	93	80	85	83	84
50	5. Ability to contribute to the cost effectiveness of treatment by collection and analysis of data on medicines' use.	58	59	95	67	69	58	68

Ranking scores were calculated (frequency rank 3 + frequency rank 4) as % of total frequency; this represents the percentage of respondents that considered a given competence as "obligatory". Competences in bold are those receiving a mean score >80%, i.e., 8/10 respondents considered these competences as "obligatory".

References

1. The PHAR-QA Project: Quality Assurance in European Pharmacy Education and Training. Available online: http://www.phar-qa.eu (accessed on 25 May 2016).
2. Atkinson, J.; de Paepe, K.; Sánchez Pozo, A.; Rekkas, D.; Volmer, D.; Hirvonen, J.; Bozic, B.; Skowron, A.; Mircioiu, C.; Marcincal, A.; et al. The PHAR-QA project: Competency framework for pharmacy practice—First steps, the results of the European network Delphi round 1. *Pharmacy* **2015**, *3*, 307–329. [CrossRef]
3. The EU Directive 2013/55/EU on the Recognition of Professional Qualifications. Available online: http://eur-lex.europa.eu/LexUriServ/LexUriServ.do?uri=OJ:L:2005:255:0022:0142:EN:PDF (accessed on 25 May 2016).
4. European Commission. The High Level Group on the Modernisation of Higher Education: Report to the European Commission. 2013. Available online: http://bookshop.europa.eu/en/high-level-group-on-the-modernisation-of-higher-education-pbNC0113156/ (accessed on 14 September 2016).
5. Landeta, J. Current validity of the Delphi method in social sciences. *Technol. Forecast. Soc. Chang.* **2006**, *73*, 467–482. [CrossRef]
6. The PHARMINE (Pharmacy Education in Europe) Consortium. Work Programme 3: Final Report Identifying and Defining Competences for Pharmacists. Available online: http://www.pharmine.org/wp-content/uploads/2014/05/PHARMINE-WP3-Final-ReportDEF_LO.pdf (accessed on 25 May 2016).
7. United Nations Industrial Development Association. Available online: http://www.unido.org/.../16959_DelphiMethod.pdf (accessed on 25 May 2016).
8. The PHAR-QA Project: Quality Assurance in European Pharmacy Education and Training. Work Package 2 "Implementation". Available online: http://www.phar-qa.eu/wp-content/uploads/2014/05/PHAR_QA_WP2_Implementation.pdf (accessed on 25 May 2016).
9. Marz, R.; Dekker, F.W.; van Schravendijk, C.; O'Flynn, S.; Ross, M.T. Tuning research competences for bologna three cycles in medicine: Report of a MEDINE2 European consensus survey. *Perpect. Med. Educ.* **2013**, *2*, 181–195. [CrossRef] [PubMed]
10. Leik, R.K. A measure of ordinal consensus. *Pac. Sociol. Rev.* **1966**, *9*, 85–90. [CrossRef]
11. Qualitative Data Systems Analysis. Qualitative Data Analysis Software (QSR). Available online: http://www.qsrinternational.com/products_nvivo.aspx (accessed on 25 May 2016).
12. Smith, A.E.; Humphreys, M.S. Evaluation of unsupervised semantic mapping of natural language with Leximancer concept mapping. *Behav. Res. Methods* **2006**, *38*, 262–279. [CrossRef] [PubMed]
13. How to Calculate Sample Size in Surveymonkey®. Available online: https://www.surveymonkey.com/mp/sample-size/ (accessed on 25 May 2016).
14. Atkinson, J.; de Paepe, K.; Sánchez Pozo, A.; Rekkas, D.; Volmer, D.; Hirvonen, J.; Bozic, B.; Skowron, A.; Mircioiu, C.; Marcincal, A.; et al. Does the subject of the pharmacy degree course influence the community pharmacist's views on competences for practice? *Pharmacy* **2015**, *3*, 12. [CrossRef]
15. Atkinson, J.; de Paepe, K.; Sánchez Pozo, A.; Rekkas, D.; Volmer, D.; Hirvonen, J.; Bozic, B.; Skowron, A.; Mircioiu, C.; Marcincal, A.; et al. How do European pharmacy students rank competences for practice? *Pharmacy* **2016**, *4*, 8. [CrossRef]
16. Atkinson, J.; Rombaut, B. The 2011 PHARMINE report on pharmacy and pharmacy education in the European Union. *Pharm. Pract. (Granada)* **2011**, *9*, 169–187. [CrossRef] [PubMed]
17. Atkinson, J.; de Paepe, K.; Sánchez Pozo, A.; Rekkas, D.; Volmer, D.; Hirvonen, J.; Bozic, B.; Skowron, A.; Mircioiu, C.; Marcincal, A.; et al. What is a pharmacist: Opinions of pharmacy department academics and community pharmacists on competences required for pharmacy practice. *Pharmacy* **2016**, *4*, 12. [CrossRef]
18. Association for Dental Education in Europe. Available online: http://www.adee.org/ (accessed on 25 May 2016).
19. Antoniou, S.; Webb, D.G.; Mcrobbie, D.; Davies, J.G.; Bates, I.P. A controlled study of the general level framework: Results of the South of England competency study. *Pharm. Educ.* **2005**, *5*, 201–207. [CrossRef]
20. Winslade, N.E.; Tamblyn, R.M.; Taylor, L.K.; Schuwirth, L.W.T.; van der Vleuten, C.P.M. Integrating performance assessment, maintenance of competence, and continuing professional development of community pharmacists. *Am. J. Pharm. Educ.* **2007**, *71*, 1–9. [CrossRef]

21. Stupans, I.; McAllister, S.; Clifford, R.; Hughes, J.; Krasse, I.; March, G.; Owen, S.; Woulf, J. Nationwide collaborative development of learning outcomes and exemplar standards for Australian pharmacy programmes. *Int. J. Pharm. Pract.* **2014**, *24*, 1–9. [CrossRef] [PubMed]
22. Box, G.E.P. Non-normality and tests on variances. *Biometrika* **1953**, *40*, 318–335. [CrossRef]
23. Ramia, E.; Salameh, P.; Btaiche, I.F.; Saa, A.H. Mapping and assessment of personal and professional development skills in a pharmacy curriculum. *BMC Med. Educ.* **2016**, *16*, 19. [CrossRef] [PubMed]

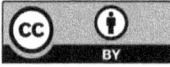

Article

What is a Pharmacist: Opinions of Pharmacy Department Academics and Community Pharmacists on Competences Required for Pharmacy Practice

Jeffrey Atkinson [1,*], Kristien de Paepe [2], Antonio Sánchez Pozo [3], Dimitrios Rekkas [4], Daisy Volmer [5], Jouni Hirvonen [6], Borut Bozic [7], Agnieska Skowron [8], Constantin Mircioiu [9], Annie Marcincal [10], Andries Koster [11], Keith Wilson [12], Chris van Schravendijk [13] and Jamie Wilkinson [14]

[1] Pharmacolor Consultants Nancy, 12 rue de Versigny, Villers 54600, France
[2] Pharmacy Faculty, Vrije Universiteit Brussel, Laarbeeklaan 103, Brussels 1090, Belgium; kdepaepe@vub.ac.be
[3] Faculty of Pharmacy, University of Granada (UGR), Campus Universitario de la Cartuja s/n, Granada 18701, Spain; sanchezp@ugr.es
[4] School of Pharmacy, National and Kapodistrian University Athens, Panepistimiou 30, Athens 10679, Greece; rekkas@pharm.uoa.gr
[5] Pharmacy Faculty, University of Tartu, Nooruse 1, Tartu 50411, Estonia; daisy.volmer@ut.ee
[6] Pharmacy Faculty, University of Helsinki, Yliopistonkatu 4, P.O. Box 33-4, Helsinki 00014, Finland; jouni.hirvonen@helsinki.fi
[7] Faculty of Pharmacy, University of Ljubljana, Askerceva cesta 7, Ljubljana 1000, Slovenia; Borut.Bozic@ffa.uni-lj.si
[8] Pharmacy Faculty, Jagiellonian University, UL, Golebia 24, Krakow 31-007, Poland; askowron@cm-uj.krakow.pl
[9] Pharmacy Faculty, University of Medicine and Pharmacy "Carol Davila" Bucharest, Dionisie Lupu 37, Bucharest 020021, Romania; constantin.mircioiu@yahoo.com
[10] European Association of Faculties of Pharmacy, Faculty of Pharmacy, Université de Lille 2, Lille 59000, France; annie.marcincal@pharma.univ-lille2.fr
[11] European Association of Faculties of Pharmacy, Dept. Pharmaceutical Sciences, Utrecht University, PO Box 80082, Utrecht 3508 TB, The Netherlands; A.S.Koster@uu.nl
[12] Applied Health Research Unit, School of Life and Health Sciences, Aston University, Birmingham B4 7ET, UK; k.a.wilson@aston.ac.uk
[13] MEDINE2, Medical Faculty, Vrije Universiteit Brussel, Laarbeeklaan 103, Brussels 1090, Belgium; chrisvs@vub.ac.be
[14] Pharmaceutical Group of the European Union (PGEU), Rue du Luxembourg 19, Brussels 1000, Belgium; j.wilkinson@pgeu.eu
* Correspondence: jeffrey.atkinson@univ-lorraine.fr; Tel./Fax: +33-383-27-37-03

Academic Editor: Yvonne Perrie
Received: 26 November 2015; Accepted: 22 January 2016; Published: 1 February 2016

Abstract: This paper looks at the opinions of 241 European academics (who provide pharmacy education), and of 258 European community pharmacists (who apply it), on competences for pharmacy practice. A proposal for competences was generated by a panel of experts using Delphi methodology. Once finalized, the proposal was then submitted to a large, European-wide community of academics and practicing pharmacists in an additional Delphi round. Academics and community pharmacy practitioners recognized the importance of the notion of patient care competences, underlining the nature of the pharmacist as a specialist of medicines. The survey revealed certain discrepancies. Academics placed substantial emphasis on research, pharmaceutical technology, regulatory aspects of quality, *etc.*, but these were ranked much lower by community pharmacists who concentrated more on patient care competences. In a sub-analysis of the data, we evaluated how perceptions may have changed since the 1980s and the introduction of the notions of competence and pharmaceutical care. This was done by splitting both groups into respondents < 40 and > 40 years old.

Results for the subgroups were essentially statistically the same but with some different qualitative tendencies. The results are discussed in the light of the different conceptions of the professional identity of the pharmacist.

Keywords: education; academic; practice

---

1. Introduction

There have been a number of changes in pharmacy education over the past 20 years starting firstly with the introduction of the concept of "competence for practice". In 1974 there were two publications in pharmacy education with the word "competence" in the title, in 2013 there were 66 [1]. Numerous frameworks have been proposed for the development and monitoring of pharmacy practice based such competence frameworks [2–5]. Several studies have shown that such competence frameworks can be successfully used to improve performance in community pharmacists [6,7]. However, little attention has been paid to the use of, and attitudes to, competence frameworks in pre-graduate, pre-registration university education. Therefore, in order to assess the relevance of pharmacy competencies, this study used the PHAR-QA "Quality Assurance in European Pharmacy Education and Training" [8] project to look at the attitudes of academics and practicing community pharmacists to the competences required for pharmacy practice.

A second change in pharmacy education over the past 20 years concerns the notion of pharmaceutical care. Pharmaceutical care is the responsible provision of drug therapy for the purpose of achieving outcomes that improve a patient's quality of life. It is englobed in a wider notion of patient care that refers to services rendered by healthcare professionals, and non-professionals under their supervision, for the benefit of the patient.

The number of articles published that have "pharmaceutical care" in the title has risen from one in 1960 to 210 in 2008 (see reference to Web of Science cited previously). This rise is similar to the rise in the interest in the notion of competence described in the previous paragraph. In a *post-hoc* sub-analysis, therefore, we looked at attitudes to competences in age sub-groups (< 40 and > 40 years old). It could be expected that the younger age subgroup will have been much more exposed to the changes outlined above than the older age subgroup.

2. Experimental Section

To evaluate academics' attitudes to competences we asked academics in European pharmacy departments to rank 68 competences for pharmacy practice. Results were compared to those obtained from practicing community pharmacists.

The numbers of respondents are statistically representative of the overall European populations (academics 10,000, community pharmacists 400,000 [9]). Respondents came from 36 different countries and although not representing a homogenous population, it was a representative selection including all significant subgroups (age, profession, region, *etc.*).

The methodology employed has been described in detail elsewhere (PHAR-QA reference cited above). The main steps are shown in Table 1.

In order to check for any possible evolution in attitudes, in a sub-analysis we compared results from 2 different age subgroups: < 40 and > 40 years of age. It is to be expected that the younger age subgroup would have been more exposed to the introduction of the concepts of competence and patient care than the older age subgroup.

GraphPad software was used for statistical analysis (ref).

Table 1. The PHAR-QA "Quality Assurance in European Pharmacy Education and Training" study methodology.

Step	Phase
1	A competence framework based on published frameworks for healthcare specialists was produced by 3 rounds of a Delphi process with an expert panel consisting of the authors of this paper, 10/13 of whom practice as pharmacists (in addition to their academic employment).
2	The competences for practice produced after the 3rd Delphi round, were ranked by a large, European-wide population of academics and community pharmacists using the PHAR-QA *surveymonkey* [10] questionnaire. Respondents came from 36/49 countries of the European Higher Education Area [11].
3	The first 6 questions were on the profile of the respondent (age, duration of practice, country of residence, current occupation (academic, community pharmacist)).
4	Questions 7 through 19 asked respondents to rank 68 competences arranged in 13 clusters of (see annex). Questions in clusters 7 (numbering succeeding the 6th question of the responder profile) through 11 were concerned with personal competences, and in clusters 12 through 19 with patient care competences.
5	Respondents were asked to rank the proposals for competences on a 4-point Likert scale: 1. Not important = Can be ignored; 2. Quite important = Valuable but not obligatory; 3. Very important = Obligatory, with exceptions depending upon field of pharmacy practice; 4. Essential = Obligatory. There was also a "cannot rank" possibility as well as the possibility of leaving an answer blank.
6	Ranking scores were calculated as (frequency rank 3 + frequency rank 4) as % of total frequency; this represents the percentage of respondents that considered a given competence as "obligatory". This calculation is based on that used by the MEDINE (*Medical Education in Europe*) consortium that ranked the competences for medical practice [12].
7	Leik ordinal consensus [13] was calculated as an indication of the dispersion of the data. Responses for consensus were arbitrarily classified as: < 0.2 poor, 0.21–0.4 fair, 0.41–0.6 moderate, 0.61–0.8 substantial, > 0.81 good, as in the MEDINE study.
8	The statistical significance of differences amongst groups was estimated from the chi-square test on the ranking frequencies; a significance level of 5% was chosen.
9	Respondents could also comment on their ranking. An attempt was made to analyze comments using the NVivo10 program [14] for the semi-quantitative analysis of unstructured data. In this case, the numbers were too small to draw significant conclusions (results not shown).

3. Results and Discussion

The overall rankings by academics and community pharmacists, given in Table 2, were similar.

Table 2. Overall distribution (*n* = 68 competences) of rankings by academics and community pharmacists.

Ranks	Academics		Community Pharmacists	
Number of respondents	241		258	
Theoretical number of replies	16,388 (= 241 respondents × 68 competences)		17,544 (= 258 × 68)	
Rank	Number	%	Number	%
4	5821	38.6	6643	37.9
3	6005	39.6	6002	34.2
2	2982	19.7	3076	17.5
1	366	4.6	608	3.5
Cannot rank + blanks	1214	8.0	1215	6.9
Score (%)	= ((5821 + 6005)/15,174) × 100) = 77.9		= [(6643 + 6002)/16,3029] × 100 = 77.4	
Leik ordinal consensus	0.58		0.55	

Seven to eight percent of respondents in both groups were not able to rank all competences. This suggests that the vast majority of respondents considered they had sufficient experience to reply to all the questions asked.

As judged from the Leik ordinal consensus values, dispersion was low. Leik ordinal consensus for rankings of individual competences ranged from 0.51 to 0.68 for academics, and from 0.42 to 0.71 for community pharmacists. This suggests that opinions in both groups were relatively homogeneous, and that subgroups with distributions of responses concerning the 68 competences significantly different from that of the overall group do not exist. Similar values for ordinal consensus were reported by the MEDINE "Medical Education in Europe" consortium. It further suggests that there are no differences between age subgroups.

Scores for individual competences, given in Table 3, differed.

Table 3. Ranking of competences (score of validated competences as important (rank 3 or 4), %) by academics and community pharmacists (*n*: sequential numbering).

Cluster	*n*	Competence	Academics	Community Pharmacists
Cluster 7. Personal competences: learning and knowledge.	1	Ability to identify learning needs and to learn independently (including continuous professional development (CPD)).	93.7	89.8
	2	Analysis: ability to apply logic to problem solving, evaluating pros and cons and following up on the solution found.	94.5	91.1
	3	Synthesis: capacity to gather and critically appraise relevant knowledge and to summarize the key points.	92.8	87.9
	4	**Capacity to evaluate scientific data in line with current scientific and technological knowledge.**	87.3	75.8
	5	Ability to interpret preclinical and clinical evidence-based medical science and apply the knowledge to pharmaceutical practice.	81.2	75.9
	6	**Ability to design and conduct research using appropriate methodology.**	65.4	40.2
	7	Ability to maintain current knowledge of relevant legislation and codes of pharmacy practice.	86.3	91.7
Cluster 8. Personal competences: values.	8	Demonstrate a professional approach to tasks and human relations.	91.5	94.5
	9	Demonstrate the ability to maintain confidentiality.	92.3	95.3
	10	**Take full personal responsibility for patient care and other aspects of one's practice.**	88.3	94.8
	11	Inspire the confidence of others in one's actions and advice.	83.8	88.8
	12	Demonstrate high ethical standards.	95.3	95.2
Cluster 9. Personal competences: communication and organizational skills.	13	Effective communication skills (both orally and written).	93.5	94.8
	14	Effective use of information technology.	83.8	86.1
	15	Ability to work effectively as part of a team.	83.3	89.2
	16	Ability to identify and implement legal and professional requirements relating to employment (e.g., for pharmacy technicians) and to safety in the workplace.	77.9	81.0
	17	Ability to contribute to the learning and training of staff.	79.6	82.5
	18	**Ability to design and manage the development processes in the production of medicines.**	60.0	43.2
	19	Ability to identify and manage risk and quality of service issues.	76.1	79.2
	20	Ability to identify the need for new services.	61.8	64.5
	21	Ability to communicate in English and/or locally relevant languages.	79.6	74.1
	22	Ability to evaluate issues related to quality of service.	71.0	77.9
	23	**Ability to negotiate, understand a business environment and develop entrepreneurship.**	46.4	64.1

Table 3. *Cont.*

Cluster	n	Competence	Academics	Community Pharmacists
Cluster 10. Personal competences: knowledge of different areas of the science of medicines.	24	Plant and animal biology.	31.1	39.3
	25	Physics.	25.6	21.7
	26	General and inorganic chemistry.	45.6	43.9
	27	**Organic and medicinal/pharmaceutical chemistry.**	80.2	66.0
	28	**Analytical chemistry.**	60.0	41.9
	29	General and applied biochemistry (medicinal and clinical).	74.2	68.8
	30	**Anatomy and physiology; medical terminology.**	75.8	88.7
	31	Microbiology.	67.0	72.2
	32	Pharmacology including pharmacokinetics.	95.6	94.7
	33	Pharmacotherapy and pharmaco-epidemiology.	92.5	94.3
	34	**Pharmaceutical technology including analyses of medicinal products.**	89.0	62.0
	35	Toxicology.	84.4	74.0
	36	Pharmacognosy.	52.9	66.5
	37	Legislation and professional ethics.	88.8	89.5
Cluster 11. Personal competences: understanding of industrial pharmacy.	38	**Current knowledge of design, synthesis, isolation, characterization and biological evaluation of active substances.**	57.5	41.7
	39	**Current knowledge of good manufacturing practice (GMP) and of good laboratory practice (GLP).**	75.4	59.4
	40	**Current knowledge of European directives on qualified persons (QPs).**	59.2	43.7
	41	**Current knowledge of drug registration, licensing and marketing.**	72.1	55.7
	42	Current knowledge of good clinical practice (GCP).	68.2	64.5
Cluster 12. Patient care competences: patient consultation and assessment.	43	Ability to perform and interpret medical laboratory tests.	65.3	65.5
	44	Ability to perform appropriate diagnostic or physiological tests to inform clinical decision making e.g., measurement of blood pressure.	64.5	73.6
	45	Ability to recognize when referral to another member of the healthcare team is needed because a potential clinical problem is identified (pharmaceutical, medical, psychological or social).	89.1	91.7
Cluster 13. Patient care competences: need for drug treatment	46	Retrieval and interpretation of relevant information on the patient's clinical background.	79.3	84.0
	47	Retrieval and interpretation of an accurate and comprehensive drug history if and when required.	89.4	91.5
	48	Identification of non-adherence and implementation of appropriate patient intervention.	85.8	86.8
	49	Ability to advise to physicians and—in some cases—prescribe medication.	80.7	87.6
Cluster 14. Patient care competences: drug interactions.	50	Identification, understanding and prioritization of drug–drug interactions at a molecular level (e.g., use of codeine with paracetamol).	91.8	91.6
	51	Identification, understanding, and prioritization of drug–patient interactions, including those that preclude or require the use of a specific drug (e.g., trastuzumab for treatment of breast cancer in women with HER2 overexpression).	87.7	89.7
	52	Identification, understanding, and prioritization of drug–disease interactions (e.g., NSAIDs in heart failure).	94.5	96.6
Cluster 15. Patient care competences: provision of drug product.	53	**Familiarity with the bio-pharmaceutical, pharmacodynamic and pharmacokinetic activity of a substance in the body.**	90.8	81.2
	54	Supply of appropriate medicines taking into account dose, correct formulation, concentration, administration route and timing.	96.3	94.9
	55	Critical evaluation of the prescription to ensure that it is clinically appropriate and legal.	94.1	94.0
	56	Familiarity with the supply chain of medicines and the ability to ensure timely flow of drug products to the patient.	78.6	84.6
	57	Ability to manufacture medicinal products that are not commercially available.	69.0	60.5

Table 3. *Cont.*

Cluster	n	Competence	Academics	Community Pharmacists
Cluster 16. Patient care competences: patient education.	58	Promotion of public health in collaboration with other actors in the healthcare system.	75.1	82.6
	59	Provision of appropriate lifestyle advice on smoking, obesity, *etc.*	71.0	80.9
	60	Provision of appropriate advice on resistance to antibiotics and similar public health issues.	89.4	93.1
Cluster 17. Patient care competences: provision of information and service.	61	Ability to use effective consultations to identify the patient's need for information.	81.1	90.9
	62	Provision of accurate and appropriate information on prescription medicines.	89.3	94.4
	63	Provision of informed support for patients in selection and use of non-prescription medicines for minor ailments (e.g., cough remedies...).	89.4	94.0
Cluster 18. Patient care competences: monitoring of drug therapy.	64	Identification and prioritization of problems in the management of medicines in a timely manner and with sufficient efficacy to ensure patient safety.	87.9	93.0
	65	Ability to monitor and report to all concerned in a timely manner, and in accordance with current regulatory guidelines on Good Pharmacovigilance Practices (GVPs), Adverse Drug Events and Reactions (ADEs and ADRs).	80.9	83.4
	66	Undertaking of a critical evaluation of prescribed medicines to confirm that current clinical guidelines are appropriately applied.	81.6	80.6
Cluster 19. Patient care competences: evaluation of outcomes.	67	Assessment of outcomes on the monitoring of patient care and follow-up interventions.	73.7	79.0
	68	Evaluation of cost effectiveness of treatment	57.7	61.2

Notes: Competences in bold are those showing a statistically significant difference in distribution of rankings between groups (chi-square, $p < 0.05$).

Both groups scored high for patient care competences (clusters 12–19). For competences linked to drug research, development and production (clusters 7 and 11), results differed.

In cluster 7 (learning and knowledge), ranks were high (> 80% for 6 out of 7 competences). Scores were lower for competence 6 (ability to design and conduct research using appropriate methodology) and fell to 40% for community pharmacists. The latter proved to be more attached to competencies connected with patient care, though this domain is less well defined and is missing from the European directive. It is also susceptible to very different interpretations from one country to another. Academics scored higher for competences related to science and research, *i.e.*, competence 4 (capacity to evaluate scientific data in line with current scientific and technological knowledge) and competence 6 (research).

For cluster 7, community pharmacists posted seven comments. This represented 0.4% of the potential total number of comments (= 258 community pharmacists × 7 propositions in cluster 7). Comments on other propositions were equally low. Comments on cluster 7 concerned the practicality of doing research *"not always practical in a busy community setting"*. Other points raised concerned the access to scientific information from reliable sources *"preselection of the new scientific information by an official institute of continuing education is necessary"* and *"get essential information from reliable sources"*. Academics posted 12 comments (0.7% of potential total) often along the same lines *"impossible for a clinical practitioner to keep up to date with even a small area of therapeutics"* and *"they are able to find synthesised forms of data (meta-analysis, systematic reviews) from trustworthy sources"*. Academics suggested that research concerned advanced studies *"important for more scientifically oriented pharmacists (Ph.D. students)"*.

In cluster 8 (values) academics scored competence 10 (responsibility for patient care) lower than did community pharmacists (88 *versus* 95%). This may be an indication of the lesser weight academics give to patient care. Albeit one academic commented *"I consider a professional approach to patients and their care as the absolute priority"*. Overall there were eight comments from academics and four from community pharmacists. One community pharmacist commented in relation to taking responsibility *"highly depends on how much information we have on patients"*. Other limitations were raised such as that from an academic *"pharmacists can't take responsibility of patient's medication; in Finland this belongs to doctors*". Another academic suggested that pharmacists should be able "*whistle-blow and call out poor practice of others*".

For two competences in cluster 9 (communication and organization) scores for academics and community pharmacists were substantially different. For competence 18 (production of medicines) academics score relatively high (60%), whereas less than half of community pharmacists (43%) considered this important. Scores for competence 23 (entrepreneurship) were the opposite with academics at 46% and community pharmacists at 64%. Comments centered on competence 18 "*no production of medicines, only dispensing*", and 21 (communication in English) "*knowledge of English not essential, knowledge of local language is essential*".

Cluster 10 ("competences" 24–37) on the science of medicines was included because the EU Directive [15] lists these 14 subject areas. These are not competences as such but foundations of competences [16]. The inclusion of these subjects provoked substantial misunderstanding with low scores for "competences" concerned with biology (24) and physics (25). Chemistry and analytical chemistry (27 and 28), and pharmaceutical technology (34) were ranked much higher by academics than by community pharmacists. Pharmacology (32) and pharmacotherapy (33) received scores >90% from both academics and community pharmacists.

Cluster 10 received the most comments—11 from academics and eight from community pharmacists. Comments from academics centered on:

- Subjects

    - "*the heart of the job is human biology and physiopathology*"
    - *Subjects to be added:*

        - *pharmaceutical care*
        - *clinical pharmacy*
        - *basic clinical knowledge*
        - *physiopathology*
        - *social sciences*
        - *statistics*

- Level and job profile

    - "*they should also have a background in sciences in general*"
    - "*differences may be in the level of knowledge for particular field on the way of professional specialization, not for the pharmacist at the beginning of the career*"
    - "*depends if we have to do with a pharmacist in hospital, industry, academy, government or local pharmacies*"

Comments from community pharmacists centered on:

- *Subjects to be added:*

    - *Pharmaceutical care*
    - *business administration*

- Level and job profile

    - "*being a pharmacist you need the basic knowledge of all the above area. Having a speciality will be important depending the sector you are going to practice*"
    - "*all answers refer to daily work in community pharmacy*"

Scores for competences in cluster 11 (industrial pharmacy) were high for academics (< 75%), but lower for community pharmacists (< 65%). There were marked differences e.g., for competence 41 (drug registration): academics 72%, community pharmacists 56%. Comments centered on job profile, with, for example, from academics: *"not really the daily preoccupation of most pharmacists"*, *"some points are essential for pharmacist in pharmaceutical industry, research and development, but it is of little importance for other pharmacists"*, and from community pharmacists *"it's not my job"*. Comments from academics raised the point that all pharmacists should have knowledge of pharmaceutical production as a basis for community practice, e.g., *"must be able to understand the security reasons behind withdrawals to explain them"*. There was some confusion regarding competence 42 (good clinical practice), some applying this to the drug research and development process, and others to community pharmacy practice.

Scores were generally high for clusters 12–19 with only one difference between academics and community pharmacists. This was for competence 53 (familiarity with the bio-pharmaceutical, pharmacodynamic and pharmacokinetic activity of a substance in the body) with academics scoring higher than community pharmacists.

Comments concerned aspects such as diagnosis (competence 44) "one of the challenges that we have come across with extending roles for pharmacists relates to body contact tests and invasive tests. Should these be covered?" Other comments concerned prescription "I would regard it as essential to be able to advise physicians, but currently it is not within the scope of practice for pharmacists to prescribe."

There were also comments on the level at which specific competence should be taught—*"competences in basic drug contraindications (drug-disease interactions) and knowledge of molecular mechanism of drug-drug interactions must be excellent already when the student finishes the university. Clinical relevance of drug-related problems plus conditions contributing to clinically significant drug-drug interactions, side effects, etc. should be trained on postgraduate level."*

Scores for competence 57 (manufacture of products not commercially available) were low. Comments centered on the fact that this activity has almost disappeared in most EU countries given the introduction of stringent regulations on GMP: *"manufacturing medicinal production is well under way of near prohibition, with stringent regulations to insure GMP. Both a good point and a bad point, as this means higher quality and controllability, but near industrial manufacturing units in a few selected drugstores, and a specific class of pharmacists."*

This low score and that for cluster 11 reveals a low awareness amongst community pharmacists that pharmacists are "medicines specialists" involved in the whole drug life cycle from R&D, through production, quality assurance, registration, patient care, pharmaco-economics and post marketing studies. This is not good for the pharmacy profession. Taken to extremes it may be concluded—based on the opinion of community pharmacists—that there is no need to employ pharmacists in the medicines industry.

Scores for cluster 16 (patient education) were high. Academics commented that *"pharmacists have a key role in offering public health/healthy living advice"* with the proviso that *"general information on diet or exercise is important but the specific recommendations for the patient should be made by the experts in those areas (f. ex. dietician or physiotherapist)."*

Scores for cluster 17 (provision of information and service) were high. Comments centered on *"pharmacist should also provide information about medical devices and other items available in the pharmacy"*, and *"need to ensure all information and products are evidence-based and appropriate for that patient."*

Scores for cluster 18 (monitoring of drug therapy) were high. Academics commented that *"safety and effectiveness are paramount—ensuring we learn from medication errors, post-marketing surveillance and demonstrate clinical effectiveness."*

Scores for cluster 19 (evaluation of outcomes) were low. Academics commented that these competences were in the domain of clinical or hospital pharmacy.

There were several general comments on methodology, for example, on the use of idiomatic English and phraseology. The construction of proposals with two or more points raised in one question (e.g., for competence 23) also clouded the issue. These and other comments on practicalities have been taken into consideration in the production of the revised version of the questionnaire.

Finally, comments throughout pointed to the esoteric nature of certain competences and the need for recognition of specialization.

Concerning the age group sub-analysis, the scores for the age subgroups of academics are given in Figure 1.

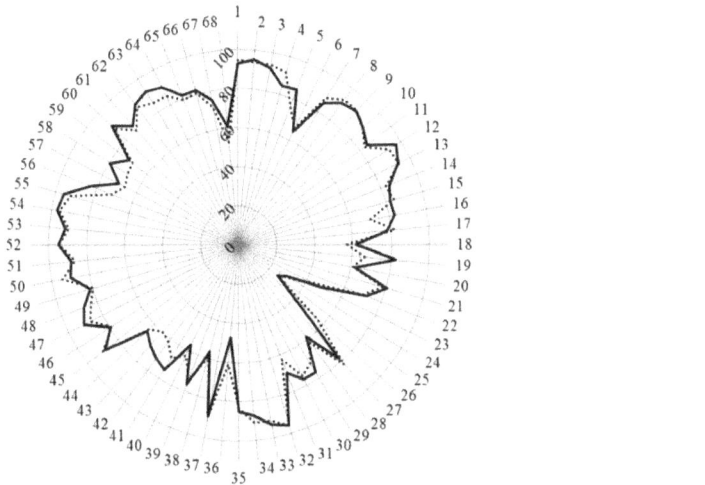

Figure 1. Scores (%) for rankings of competences by academics over 40 (*n* = 144, solid line) and under 40 (*n* = 97, dotted line).

Chi-square revealed one difference only—that for competence 19 (quality of service) where academics over 40 scored higher than those under 40. For competences 6, 18, 28, 38, and 40 where there were major differences between academics and community pharmacists (see above), there were no significant differences between the two age subgroups of academics. Overall these data suggest that there is no evolution in the opinions, concerning the topics mentioned, of academics with age. Furthermore the fact of having been exposed during their own education to concepts such as "pharmaceutical care" and "competence for practice" (*i.e.*, < 40 years of age) does not appear to influence their rankings for patient care competences. Carrying on from this, it can be suggested that the differences between academics and community pharmacists noted previously is not a question of age.

The above results can be understood very negatively, *i.e.*, what academics learned 25 years ago they consider is still valid. The study is cross-sectional and measures what academics > 40 think today, not what they thought 25 years ago. There is probably no difference with age due to evolution of opinions according to the state of the art in the field: evidence-based pharmacy influences opinions of academics regardless of age.

The scores for the age subgroups of community pharmacists are given in Figure 2.

Chi-square revealed one difference only—that for competence 41 (drug registration) where community pharmacists under 40 scored higher than those over 40; otherwise there were no statistically significant differences. It is to be noted that for the 7–17 competences concerning values and communication, as well as in the group 60–65 concerning again the relation with patients, young pharmacists were somewhat less enthusiastic than their elder colleagues, in spite of the clear movement of community pharmacy practice in this direction. For competences 6, 18, 28, 38, and 40 where there were major differences between community pharmacists and academics (see above), there were no significant differences between the two age subgroups of community pharmacists. Overall these data suggest that there is no evolution in the opinions of community pharmacists with age.

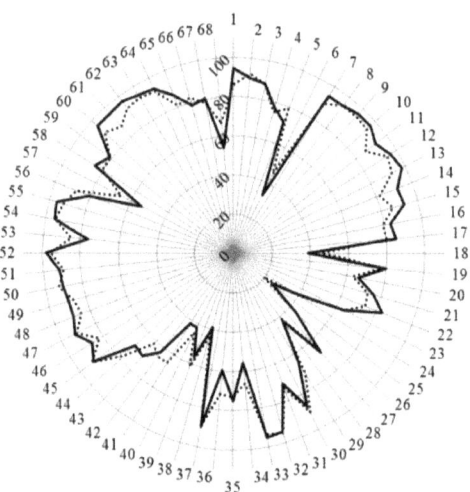

Figure 2. Scores (%) for rankings of competences by community pharmacists over 40 (*n* = 110, solid line) and under 40 (*n* = 148, dotted line).

4. Conclusions

While surveys of pharmacist perceptions of competence standards have been carried out elsewhere, for example in Thailand [17], to our knowledge, this is the first such survey on a large scale in Europe, although a similar study on competences for medical doctors has been published by MEDINE. Many techniques can be used to identify competencies for practice. Grussing [18] has suggested using multiple methods such as generation by a panel, validation by practitioner surveys or by job analysis. We used the first two of these: generation of a proposal for competences by a panel of experts followed by validation on a large, European-wide scale. We suggest that this double approach strengthens the recommendations of the PHAR-QA consortium.

The general message of this PHAR-QA study is that both academics and community pharmacist recognize the importance of the notion of patient care, as reflected by the high scores for patient care competences. The rankings and the comments underline the nature of the pharmacist as a specialist of medicines, capable making critical evaluations on therapy, and advising the patient as to the best use of medicines.

Community pharmacists gave low scores to drug research, development and production, in spite of the fact that, historically, these domains are the building blocks of pharmacy. As far as research is concerned, this low score is not reflected in the opinions of other healthcare professionals. Thus in the MEDINE2 study on competences for medical practice, medical doctors thought that *"learning outcomes related both to 'using research' and 'doing research' should be core components of medical curricula"*.

In other studies the message is more equivocal. In the Elvey *et al.* [19] study (Who do you Think You Are? Pharmacists' Perceptions of Their Professional Identity), the authors asked professional pharmacists to give their opinions on nine possible professional identities. They concluded that "While the scientist was the strongest professional identity to emerge it nevertheless seemed to overlap and compete with other professional identities … "

This leads on to the question asked by Waterfield [20]: *"Is pharmacy a knowledge-based profession?"* Waterfield concludes that *"The closer integration of science and practice is another area that needs to be considered by educators as they consider the place of practice-based knowledge."* They stress the importance of the place of science in pharmacy curricula and practice. The future challenge will be to instill a sense of science-based practice into the mind of the practizing pharmacist, and this via both pre- and postgraduate (continuous professional development) education.

The PHAR-QA study raises the point of specialization in pharmacy education. The nature and depth of the subjects to be dealt with varies as a function of the orientation for a given professional practice. Several comments suggested that competences dealing with research, industrial pharmacy, and pharmaceutical technology belong to specialized, postgraduate education for industrial pharmacy. Competences related to assessment of outcomes and monitoring of patient care; these were considered to be in the domain of a hospital pharmacy specialization.

5. Perspectives

In the light of the rankings and comments, a revised version of the survey on the competence framework was produced [21]. This second round will be followed by the publication of a PHAR-QA competence framework for pharmacy practice. Using the PHAR-QA competence framework it will be possible to compare attitudes with the emphases of the same categories in current pharmacy school curricula. Thus suggestions could be made for change in such curricula to address what seems to be a shifting preference of emphasis.

The PHAR-QA competence framework could be incorporated into pharmacy education at various levels of Miller's triangle [22]. This triangle describes a conceptual, pyramidal model of the various facets of competence with four levels, from level 1 "knows" to level 4 "does". Given the low scores of most of the subject areas (cluster 10), it would appear that academics and community pharmacists do not grasp the importance of level 1 subjects as building blocks of the level 2 competences. The PHAR-QA framework could be used to develop integrated, coordinated courses that combine several subjects under a broad competence heading. Another use of the PHAR-QA competence framework could be the accreditation at level 2 "knows how". This would allow a realistic evaluation of a student's ability to synthesize different subjects into comprehensive competences. The PHAR-QA framework could also be used at the third level in the performance testing of students. Patient substitutes could present students with elements such as symptoms, prescriptions, *etc.* calling upon PHAR-QA competences to solve problems related to drug interaction and other aspects.

Acknowledgments: With the support of the Lifelong Learning program of the European Union: 527194-LLP-1-2012-1-BE-ERASMUS-EMCR. This project has been funded with support from the European Commission. This publication reflects the views only of the author; the Commission cannot be held responsible for any use that may be made of the information contained therein.

Author Contributions: Jeffrey Atkinson designed, constructed, ran and analyzed the survey and wrote the paper. Kristien De Paepe ran the PHAR-QA consortium. Constantin Mircioiu played a major role in the statistical analyses of the data. Antonio Sánchez Pozo and Dimitrios Rekkas developed the questionnaire. Antonio Sánchez Pozo, Dimitrios Rekkas, Jouni Hirvonen, Borut Bozic, Annie Marcincal and Agnieska Skowron helped with distribution of the survey. Antonio Sánchez Pozo, Daisy Volmer, Keith Wilson and Kristien De Paepe provided useful criticism and suggestions during revision of the manuscript. Chris van Schravendijk assured the contacts with MEDINE. Jamie Wilkinson helped distribute the survey.

Conflicts of Interest: The authors declare no conflict of interest.

References

1. Web of Science Database. Available online: http://apps.webofknowledge.com (accessed on 6 January 2016).
2. CoDEG (Competency Development and Evaluation Group). General Level Practice. Available online: http://www.codeg.org/frameworks/general-level-practice/ (accessed on 6 January 2016).
3. Accreditation Council for Pharmacy Education. ACPE Open Forum: Accreditation Standards 2016. Available online: http://www.aacp.org/governance/SIGS/assessment/Assessment%20Docs/AACP%202014 %20Interim%20Meeting%20%20presentation%20-%20ACPE%20Standards%202016.pdf (accessed on 6 January 2016).

4. Stupans, I.; McAllister, S.; Clifford, R.; Hughes, J.; Krass, I.; March, G.; Owen, S.; Woulfeg, J. Nationwide collaborative development of learning outcomes and exemplar standards for Australian pharmacy programmes. *Int. J. Pharm. Pract.* **2015**, *23*, 283–291. [CrossRef] [PubMed]
5. FIP/WHO. International Pharmaceutical Federation—World Health Organisation: Standards for quality of pharmacy services. Available online: https://www.fip.org/ (accessed on 6 January 2016).
6. Antoniou, S.; Webb, D.G.; Mcrobbie, D.; Davies, J.G.; Bates, I.P. A controlled study of the general level framework: Results of the South of England Competency Study. *Pharm. Educ.* **2005**, *5*, 1–8. [CrossRef]
7. Coombes, I.; Avent, M.; Cardiff, L.; Bettenay, K.; Coombes, J.; Whitfield, K.; Stokes, J.; Davies, G.; Bates, I. Improvement in pharmacist's performance facilitated by an adapted competency-based general level framework. *J. Pharm. Pract. Res.* **2010**, *40*, 111–118. [CrossRef]
8. Atkinson, J.; de Paepe, K.; Sánchez Pozo, A.; Rekkas, D.; Volmer, D.; Hirvonen, J.; Bozic, B.; Skowron, A.; Mircioiu, C.; Marcincal, A.; *et al.* The PHAR-QA Project: Competency framework for pharmacy practice—First steps, the results of the European network Delphi Round 1. *Pharmacy* **2015**, *3*, 307–329. [CrossRef]
9. PHARMINE (Pharmacy Education in Europe). Report on Work Programme 3. Available online: http://www.pharmine.org/wp-content/uploads/2014/05/PHARMINE-final-report-Lisbon-0611.pdf (accessed on 6 January 2016).
10. Survey Software, Inc. The Survey System. Available online: http://www.surveysystem.com/sscalc.htm (accessed on 6 January 2016).
11. The Bologna Process. The European Higher Education Area. Available online: http://www.ehea.info/ (accessed on 6 January 2016).
12. Marz, R.; Dekker, F.W.; Van Schravendijk, C.; O'Flynn, S.; Ross, M.T. Tuning research competences for Bologna three cycles in medicine: Report of a MEDINE2 European Consensus Survey. *Perp. Med. Educ.* **2013**, *2*, 189–195. [CrossRef] [PubMed]
13. Leik, R.K. A measure of ordinal consensus. *Pac. Soc. Rev.* **1966**, *9*, 85–90. Available online: http://www.jstor.org/stable/1388242 (accessed on 6 January 2016). [CrossRef]
14. Qualitative Data Systems Analysis. Qualitative Data Analysis Software (QSR). Available online: http://www.qsrinternational.com/products_nvivo.aspx (accessed on 6 January 2016).
15. The European Commission. The EU Directive 2013/55/EU on the Recognition of Professional Qualifications. Available online: http://eur-lex.europa.eu/LexUriServ/LexUriServ.do?uri = OJ: L:2005:255:0022:0142:EN:PDF (accessed on 6 January 2016).
16. Fernandez, N.; Dory, V.; Ste-Maris, L.-G.; Chaput, M.; Charlin, B.; Boucher, A. Varying conceptions of competence: An analysis of how health science educators define competence. *Med. Educ. Rev.* **2012**, *46*, 357–365. [CrossRef] [PubMed]
17. Maitreemit, P.; Pongcharoensuk, P.; Kapol, N.; Armstrong, E.P. Pharmacist Perceptions of New Competency Standards. Available online: http://www.pharmacypractice.org/journal/index.php/pp/article/view/207 (accessed on 6 January 2016).
18. Grussing, P.G. Education and practice: Is competency-based education closing the gap? *Am. J. Pharm. Educ.* **1984**, *48*, 117–124. [PubMed]
19. Elvey, R.; Hassell, K.; Hall, K. Who do you Think You Are? Pharmacists' Perceptions of Their Professional Identity. Available online: http://onlinelibrary.wiley.com/doi/10.1111/ijpp.12019/abstract (accessed on 6 January 2016).
20. Waterfield, J. Is pharmacy a knowledge-based profession? *Am. J. Pharm. Educ.* **2010**, *74*, 1–6. [CrossRef]
21. The PHAR-QA Survey on Competences for Pharmacy Practice: Round 2. Available online: https://www.surveymonkey.com/r/pharqa2 (accessed on 26 January 2016).
22. Miller, G.E. The assessment of clinical skills/competences/performance. *Acad. Med.* **1990**, *65*, 63–67. [CrossRef]

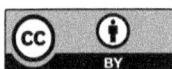

pharmacy

MDPI

Article

Hospital and Community Pharmacists' Perceptions of Which Competences Are Important for Their Practice

Jeffrey Atkinson [1,*], Antonio Sánchez Pozo [2], Dimitrios Rekkas [3], Daisy Volmer [4], Jouni Hirvonen [5], Borut Bozic [6], Agnieska Skowron [7], Constantin Mircioiu [8], Roxana Sandulovici [8], Annie Marcincal [9,10], Andries Koster [9,11], Keith A. Wilson [12], Chris van Schravendijk [13], Roberto Frontini [14,15], Richard Price [15], Ian Bates [16] and Kristien De Paepe [17]

1   Pharmacolor Consultants Nancy, 12 rue de Versigny, Villers 54600, France
2   Faculty of Pharmacy, University of Granada (UGR), Campus Universitario de la Cartuja s/n, Granada 18701, Spain; sanchezpster@gmail.com
3   School of Pharmacy, National and Kapodistrian University Athens, Panepistimiou 30, Athens 10679, Greece; rekkas@pharm.uoa.gr
4   Pharmacy Faculty, University of Tartu, Nooruse 1, Tartu 50411, Estonia; daisy.volmer@ut.ee
5   Pharmacy Faculty, University of Helsinki, Yliopistonkatu 4, P.O. Box 33-4, Helsinki 00014, Finland; jouni.hirvonen@helsinki.fi
6   Faculty of Pharmacy, University of Ljubljana, Askerceva cesta 7, Ljubljana 1000, Slovenia; Borut.Bozic@ffa.uni-lj.si
7   Pharmacy Faculty, Jagiellonian University, UL, Golebia 24, Krakow 31-007, Poland; askowron@cm-uj.krakow.pl
8   Pharmacy Faculty, University of Medicine and Pharmacy "Carol Davila" Bucharest, Dionisie Lupu 37, Bucharest 020021, Romania; constantin.mircioiu@yahoo.com (C.M.); roxana.sandulovici@yahoo.com (R.S.)
9   European Association of Faculties of Pharmacy, Department of Pharmacy, Faculty of Medicine and Surgery, University of Malta, Msida MSD 2080, Malta; annie.marcincal@univ-lille2.fr (A.M.); A.S.Koster@uu.nl (A.K.)
10   Faculty of Pharmacy, Université de Lille 2, Lille 59000, France
11   Department Pharmaceutical Sciences, Utrecht University, PO Box 80082, Utrecht 3508 TB, The Netherlands
12   Applied Health Research Unit, School of Life and Health Sciences, Aston University, Birmingham B4 7ET, UK; k.a.wilson@aston.ac.uk
13   Medical Faculty, Vrije Universiteit Brussel, Laarbeeklaan 103, Brussels 1090, Belgium; chrisvs@vub.ac.be
14   University Hospital of Leipzig, Centre for Patient Safety, Liebigstrasse 20, Leipzig 04103, Germany; roberto.frontini@medizin.uni-leipzig.de
15   European Association of Hospital Pharmacists, Rue Abbe Cuypers 3, Brussels 1040, Belgium; richard.price@eahp.eu
16   School of Pharmacy, University College London, Gower Street, London WC1E 6BT, UK; i.bates@ucl.ac.uk
17   Pharmacy Faculty, Vrije Universiteit Brussel, Laarbeeklaan 103, Brussels 1090, Belgium; kdepaepe@vub.ac.be
*   Correspondence: jeffrey.atkinson@univ-lorraine.fr; Tel./Fax: +33-383-27-37-03

Academic Editor: Yvonne Perrie
Received: 20 March 2016; Accepted: 3 June 2016; Published: 15 June 2016

Abstract: The objective of the PHAR-QA (Quality assurance in European pharmacy education and training) project was to investigate how competence-based learning could be applied to a healthcare, sectoral profession such as pharmacy. This is the first study on evaluation of competences from the pharmacists' perspective using an improved Delphi method with a large number of respondents from all over Europe. This paper looks at the way in which hospital pharmacists rank the fundamental competences for pharmacy practice. European hospital pharmacists ($n = 152$) ranked 68 competences for pharmacy practice of two types (personal and patient care), arranged into 13 clusters. Results were compared to those obtained from community pharmacists ($n = 258$). Generally, hospital and community pharmacists rank competences in a similar way. Nevertheless, differences can be detected. The higher focus of hospital pharmacists on knowledge of the different areas of science as well as on laboratory tests reflects the idea of a hospital pharmacy specialisation. The difference is also visible in the field of drug production. This is a necessary competence in hospitals with requests for drugs for rare diseases, as well as paediatric and oncologic drugs. Hospital pharmacists give entrepreneurship a lower score, but cost-effectiveness a higher one than community pharmacists. This reflects the reality of pharmacy practice where community pharmacists have to act as entrepreneurs, and hospital pharmacists are managers staying within drug budgets. The results are discussed in the light of a "hospital pharmacy" specialisation.

Keywords: education; specialisation; practice

1. Introduction

Competence-based learning is not new and is not limited to pharmacy education. The number of published articles on competence-based learning in all areas has risen from one per year in 1982 to 65 per year in 2012 [1]. We investigated how this competence-based approach could be applied to pharmacy. Thus the first objective of the PHAR-QA (Quality assurance in European pharmacy education and training) project [2] was to investigate how competence-based learning could be applied to a healthcare, sectoral profession such as pharmacy in which competences are linked to well-defined outcomes such as patient safety. The second objective of the study concerned the European nature of the pharmacy profession given that pharmacists educated and trained in a given member state have the right, under the freedom of movement directives of the European Union (EU), to practice in another member state [3]. A third objective concerned the organisation of the EU university degree course into a fundamental three-year bachelor course followed by a specialised two-year master course according to the Bologna declaration [4]. Most of the faculties of pharmacy in Europe have a five-year degree course [5]. This is an integrated, seamless model with the pharmacy "bachelor" course at a fundamental level followed by a more specialised "master" course. Here we will examine whether a case can be made for a difference between education and training in future community and hospital pharmacy master degrees.

The discussion on the existence or not of the specialisation of hospital pharmacy has several elements. Regarding work location, graduates with a pharmacy degree are employed in a variety of positions, two of the most important (in terms of numbers) being community and hospital pharmacy (Table 1). Figures for hospital pharmacists vary 10-fold from Spain to the UK. Average figures for employment of pharmacists from the 26 EU member states with university pharmacy departments, published by the PHARMINE "Pharmacy Education in Europe" consortium, were 81% in community and 5% in hospital practice [5]. World-wide figures given by the International Pharmaceutical Federation (FIP) are 55% for community and 18% for hospital practice (with large regional variation) [6]. FIP data for Europe ($n = 22$) is 7.2% of pharmacists working in a hospital, similar to the PHARMINE figure.

Table 1. Percentages of pharmacists in community and hospital practice in four European countries.

PHARMACISTS	France [7]	Germany [8]	Spain [9]	UK [10]
Community	75	81	58	72
Hospital	12	4	2	23

Regarding the education for hospital pharmacists, the PHARMINE study [5] reported that university pharmacy departments in 18/26 European countries have a traineeship in a hospital pharmacy during their 5-year course. Thus in the majority of departments the need for training in a hospital environment is recognised as an option.

Regarding the legislation for hospital pharmacists, in some European countries, the status of hospital pharmacist is officially defined by national law and the statutes of the pharmacy professional body, e.g., France, Spain, Italy, Belgium, Netherlands, Portugal, and Switzerland. However, at the European level, this is not a universal approach. In the European Union (EU), the 1985 EU directive on the profession of pharmacy [11] did not recognise any specialisations in pharmacy (although these are recognised in medicine and dentistry). The 2013 update [12] opened up the possibility for specialties of any of the seven automatically recognised professions (medicine, dentistry, veterinary, midwifery, nursing, pharmacy, architects) to be recognised via the creation of a "Common Training Framework" [13]. A CTF is a new EU tool to achieve automatic professional qualification recognition—including for specialties of pharmacy practice, such as hospital pharmacy—across EU countries.

In the light of the previous chapters, it appears, therefore, that the argument for the existence of a specialised pharmacy job description of "hospital pharmacist" different from that for other specialities such as community pharmacy, although recognised by most university pharmacy departments, lacks a clear common pan-European expression. This is a matter that the European Association of Hospital Pharmacists (EAHP) is seeking to address via a project to form a common training framework for hospital pharmacy in Europe [14].

Pharmacists working in a hospital environment represent a significant sector of practising pharmacists and the hospital pharmacist can be defined by his/her competences and tasks. Differences between hospital and community pharmacists are to be expected in several areas of practice such as patient care and pharmaceutical technology. Community pharmacists are in direct contact with patients and are councillors of ambulatory patients; treatment is frequently symptomatic, based on prescriptions and discussions with the patient, and concerns chronic illness. Hospital pharmacists, and especially clinical pharmacists, are in direct contact with medical doctors and their tasks concern mainly hospitalised patients. Changes in the treatment of hospitalised patients are frequently decided in agreement with the hospital pharmacist. Thus hospital pharmacists are more involved with the treatment starting with interpretation of laboratory tests and diagnosis. The diseases treated are acute and more severe involving complications such as microbial resistance and nosocomial infections that are often evaluated mainly by hospital pharmacists. Hospital pharmacy, however, is evolving in different areas of patient care in the hospital. First, there is a shift towards direct participation in the establishment of treatment by clinical pharmacy teams. The second shift is in the evaluation and establishment of the drug treatment of patients when they leave hospital—an activity similar to that of community pharmacy. Concerning pharmaceutical technology, there has been a shift in medicine production from compounding in pharmacies to industrial production since the 1950s [15]. Compounding in hospital pharmacies has, however, been maintained for paediatric and other specialised formulations.

A conceptual issue here is whether one defines and distinguishes between "community pharmacists" and "hospital pharmacists" on the basis of their working environment or on the basis of different tasks and different responsibilities. Making the distinction on the basis of task/responsibility analysis, as in the case here, will be more useful for curriculum development and for the discussion about differentiated study programmes. Therefore "job description" can be useful, but should not be translated as "working in a hospital." There are examples of community pharmacists working in hospitals.

Within this context, we investigated in the PHAR-QA ("*Quality Assurance in European PHARmacy Education and Training*") project [16], whether the ranking by hospital pharmacists of competences for practice is different from that of community pharmacists.

We asked community and hospital pharmacists to rank competences for pharmacy practice. Competences were essentially based on those established in the previous PHARMINE project [17] with input from the MEDINE group [18] who ran a similar project on the evaluation of competences for medical practice by medical doctors and students, and from previous competence frameworks for pharmacy practice [19,20].

This paper describes the similarities and differences between how European hospital and community pharmacists rank competences for pharmacy practice.

2. Experimental Section

Ranking data on competences for practice were obtained using the PHAR-QA *surveymonkey* [21] questionnaire that was available online from 14 February 2014 through 1 November 2014 *i.e.*, 8.5 months [22]. Respondents came from 25 EU countries.

The first six questions were on the profile of the respondent (age, duration of practice, country of residence, current occupation (hospital, community, ... pharmacist). Questions in clusters 7 through 19 asked about 68 competences for pharmacy practice (see annex). Clusters 7 through 11 were concerned with personal competences, and clusters 12 through 19 with patient care competences. The competences came mainly from PHARMINE [17], MEDINE [18] and the EU directive on sectoral professions [12].

Respondents (hospital pharmacists, $n = 152$, community pharmacists, $n = 258$) were asked to rank the proposals for competences on a four-point Likert scale:

1. Not important = Can be ignored.
2. Quite important = Valuable but not obligatory.
3. Very important = Obligatory, with exceptions depending upon field of pharmacy practice.
4. Essential = Obligatory.

There was also a "cannot rank" possibility, as well as the possibility of leaving the answer blank.

In order to evaluate the effect of age on results, two matched age subgroups were created *post hoc*: age < 40 years old or age > 40 years old. This comparison was based on age rather than duration of practice as (1) in many cases information on the duration of practice was not available (see Table 2); and (2) duration of practice would not take into account late starters.

Table 2. Duration of practice (years) in hospital and community pharmacist respondents.

Respondents	Duration of Practice (Years)						
	< 5	6–10	11–20	21–30	31–40	Did not Answer	Total
Hospital pharmacists *n* (%)	37 (24.3)	46 (30.3)	30 (19.8)	26 (17.1)	2 (1.3)	11 (7.2)	152
Community pharmacists *n* (%)	50 (19.4)	51 (19.8)	41 (15.9)	49 (19.0)	7 (2.7)	60 (23.2)	258

n: number in each category. Chi-squared test for duration of practice hospital *versus* community = 4.27, degrees of freedom = 4, $p > 0.05$.

Results are presented in the form of "scores," calculated as follows: score = (frequency rank 3 + frequency rank 4) as % of total frequency, *i.e.*, obligatory as a % of total. This calculation is based on that made by the MEDINE consortium in their study on the ranking of competences for medical practice [18]. Such scores are used for descriptive purposes only and no conclusions on statistical differences amongst groups are based on scores.

Leik ordinal consensus [23] was calculated as an indication of the dispersion of the data using an Excel spreadsheet. The original Leik paper cited gives an explicit mathematical example of the calculation of ordinal consensus. Responses for consensus were arbitrarily classified as: < 0.2 poor, 0.21–0.4 fair, 0.41–0.6 moderate, 0.61–0.8 substantial, > 0.81 good, according to the scale proposed in the MEDINE study [18].

The statistical significance of differences amongst groups was estimated from the chi-square test on the original ranking frequencies; a significance level of 5% was chosen. Statistical tests were performed using GraphPad software (Graphpad Software Inc, La Jolla, CA, USA) [24].

Respondents could also add their comments on the different clusters in a text box presented simultaneously with the questions on ranking. An attempt was made to analyse comments using the NVivo10 programme [25] and the Leximancer programme [26] for the semi-quantitative analysis of unstructured data. It was found that the numbers involved were too small to draw significant conclusions, so comments are grouped into clusters.

Ethical concerns on the research included two aspects. First was the avoidance of collecting personal data that was not relevant to the research. The second was to avoid judgement of differences amongst groups. The case of very low ranks for physics and analytical chemistry were treated as misunderstanding following a lack of sufficient clarity in the formulation of the questions. The protocol and results were analysed by the National Commission Drug Bioethics of Romania [27].

3. Results and Discussion

The distribution of numbers of respondents by duration of practice of the groups is given in Table 2.

The distributions of duration of practice were not significantly different. In both cases, most respondents had less than 20 years of experience, thus a relatively "young" population seems to be involved.

Respondents in both groups came from 25 European countries. Hospital pharmacy respondents came mainly from Spain (n = 36) and the United Kingdom (n = 28).

Table 3 shows the overall distribution of rankings by hospital and community pharmacists.

Table 3. Overall distribution (n = 68 competences) of rankings of hospital and community pharmacists.

RANKING	Hospital Pharmacists		Community Pharmacists	
Number of respondents	152		258	
Theoretical total number of replies	10,336 (=152 × 68)		17,544 (=258 × 68)	
Rank	Number	%	Number	%
4	3948	38.2	6643	37.9
3	3767	36.5	6002	34.2
2	1838	17.8	3076	17.5
1	316	3.1	608	3.5
Cannot rank + blanks	467	4.5	1215	6.9
Score (%)	= ((3948 + 3767)/9869) × 100 = 78.2		= ((6643 + 6002)/16,329) × 100 = 77.4	
Leik ordinal consensus	0.62		0.65	

Chi-square test for comparison of the distribution of ranks for hospital *versus* community pharmacists revealed a significant difference: $p < 0.05$ (degrees of freedom = 3 ((4 ranks − 1) × (2 groups − 1)).

Overall ranking by hospital pharmacists was statistically significantly higher than that by community pharmacists, though the difference was very small.

Only 4.5% (hospital) and 6.9% (community) of respondents were unable to rank competences, suggesting that both groups considered themselves sufficiently informed to reply to the questions asked, and the questions were pertinent to their ideas on practice. This is backed up by the relatively high Leik ordinal consensus values, showing that ordinal dispersion was not great. Thus subgroups do not exist. Similar values for ordinal consensus have been reported by the MEDINE consortium.

Figures 1 and 2 show the results for analysis by competences. Figure 1 shows the values for Leik ordinal consensus.

The ordinal consensus values were in most cases higher than 0.5, and similar in both groups.

Scores for the 68 competences are given in Figure 2 and in detail in table A1 in the appendix.

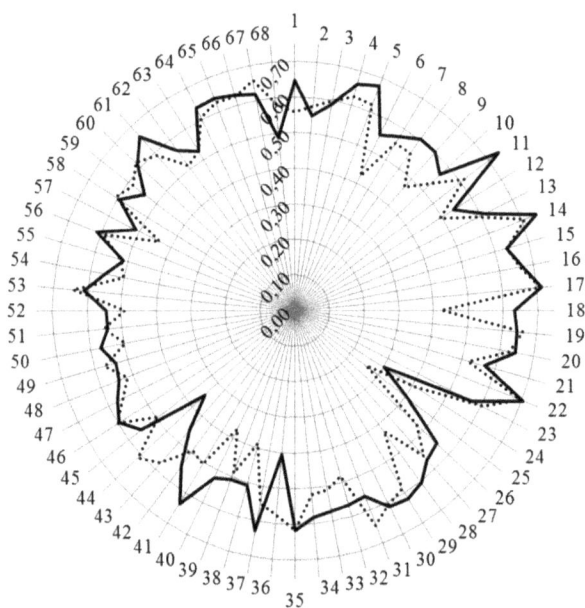

Figure 1. Leik ordinal consensus for rankings by competences for hospital and community pharmacists. Hospital pharmacists: full line; community pharmacists: dotted line.

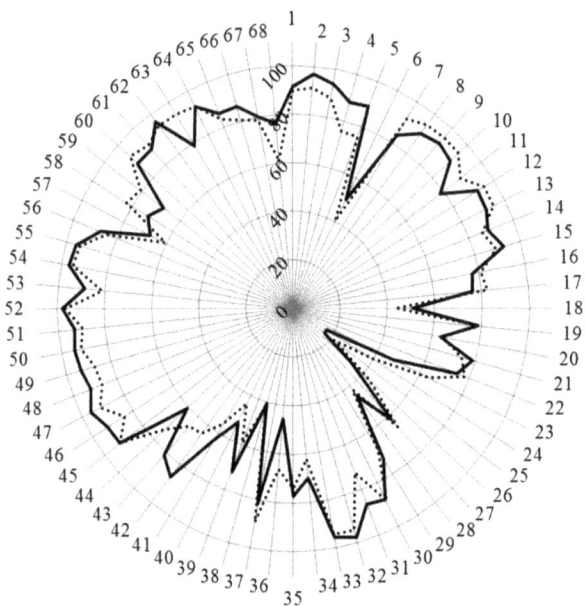

Figure 2. Scores (%) for rankings of competences for hospital and community pharmacists (results in annex). Hospital pharmacists: full line; community pharmacists: dotted line.

3.1. Cluster 7. Personal Competences: Learning and Knowledge

For the personal competences, cluster 7 "learning and knowledge" (competences 1–7), the scores of hospital pharmacists for competences relating to evaluation and interpretation of, and keeping up to date with, scientific data and evidence-based medical science were higher than those of community pharmacists. Scores for both groups were low for competence 6 related to research but were higher for hospital pharmacists. There was also lower consensus on this competence (Figure 1) showing that, especially for community pharmacists, opinion on the importance of competence in the area of research was split.

There were 32 comments made by hospital pharmacists. These represent ((32/10,336) × 100) = 0.3% of the theoretical total of possible comments. For cluster 7, there were three comments: two on research along the lines of the need for "knowledge = being aware of" rather than "ability = capable of doing." The third comment expressed sectoral concerns: "*My answers would change if I was looking just at hospital pharmacists or just community pharmacist . . . I think different skills are of varying importance depending on the sector.*" This concern was expressed elsewhere regarding other competences.

3.2. Cluster 8. Personal Competences: Values

For the personal competences, cluster 8 "values" (competences 8–12), the scores of hospital pharmacists were globally lower than those of community pharmacists, especially for those competences concerning human relations such as "inspiring confidence in one's actions" (competence 11). There were two comments from hospital pharmacists on cluster 8. The first stressed the qualities needed for interaction with other (healthcare) professionals: "*In order to collaborate with other professionals, pharmacists have to show a high degree of responsibility and knowledge.*" The second comment raised the difficulty of evaluating ethical competences: "*I have always wondered how someone can prove 'competence' of approach to human relations and high ethical standards. I would presume that these are not proven . . . *"

3.3. Cluster 9. Personal Competences: Communication and Organisational Skills

For the personal competences, cluster 9 "communication and organisation" values (competences 13–23), the scores of hospital pharmacists were similar to those of community pharmacists except for competence 23 regarding "entrepreneurship," where hospital pharmacists scored lower than community pharmacists. There were three comments on cluster 9, two expressing sectoral concerns as seen for cluster 7 above. The third concerned language issues: "*Does competency 21 relate to students from English-speaking countries only? Effective communication in the local native language is foremost, important and essential. Good written and spoken English is useful for those wishing to understand research and work at international levels and therefore I'd class this as quite important for non-English speaking countries.*"

3.4. Cluster 10. Personal Competences: Knowledge of Different Areas of the Science of Medicines

For the personal competences in cluster 10, "knowledge of the different areas of science" (competences 24–37), the scores of hospital pharmacists were similar to those of community pharmacists except for competences 24 "biology" and 36 "pharmacognosy" where scores for hospital pharmacists were lower, and competence 31 "microbiology" where scores were higher. It should be noted that consensus for competence 24 was low (Figure 1), suggesting that not all agreed on a low score. There were six comments on cluster 10, with one on sectoral concerns as noted above. Three other comments were on the relative importance of the different knowledge areas (greater importance of pharmacology, pharmaceutical technology, *etc.* and of "clinical" subjects"). One comment suggested including social sciences. One comment stressed the need to coordinate tertiary education with secondary education, thereby suggesting that several subjects listed could be dealt with in more detail and depth at the secondary level. It should be noted that cluster 10 was included because considerable emphasis has been placed in the EU directive 2013/55/EU on the recognition of professional qualifications (see above). These are not competencies as generally recognised in the educational literature, syllabus or curriculum. There is no behavioural component, or reflections of values/attitudes which are considered desirable for practice-related competencies. Knowledge of a subject is not a competence in itself but part of a competence. Competencies are generally assumed to comprise behavioural components rather than syllabus components and should be linked to scope of practice. It is the latter which is the important angle, as this is the actual link with patient care. Finally, the educational system may influence these findings, if, for example, a pharmacy student opts for a hospital, community, industry or other track. Thus different educational and training systems may introduce certain biases.

3.5. Cluster 11. Personal Competences: Understanding of Industrial Pharmacy

For the personal competences of cluster 11, "industrial pharmacy" (competences 38–42), the scores of hospital pharmacists were higher for four out of five competences relating to legislation and drug production and registration. There were two comments, one again on sectoral concerns. The second concerned the importance of EU directives (competence 40): *"The knowledge about EU legislative is crucial for the pharmacist in the EU countries. For the others—non-EU members—the EU legislative is very important as well, as there is a tendency in unification i.e., maximal improving of the pharmacy practice."* It is to be noted that the fact that competence 42, "good clinical practice," is placed within an industrial pharmacy cluster could be interpreted as meaning "good clinical practice in the clinical phase of evaluation of a new chemical entity during the drug registration procedure" rather than "good practice in the exercise of one's job." This and other ambiguous phrases were corrected in the second version of the PHAR-QA questionnaire (see the perspective section below).

Ranking of competences in the areas of research, pharmaceutical technology and industrial pharmacy (clusters 10 and 11) are also influenced by the evolution in the way in which medicines are produced. Since the 1950s, several factors have produced a shift in drug production from small-scale, artisanal compounding in pharmacies to large-scale production by the pharmaceutical industry [15]. These factors include the introduction of new drugs, such as antibiotics, vaccines, anti-hypertensives, tranquillizers and antidepressants, the research and development of which requires investment on a large, industrial scale as does the ongoing development of therapies for chronic diseases such as Alzheimer's disease, the development of biosimilars and the other products of pharmaceutical biotechnology, and the development of treatment with generic drugs [28]. Compounding has continued in specialised hospital settings including the area of sterile preparations and of paediatric therapy [29].

3.6. Cluster 12. Patient Care Competences: Patient Consultation and Assessment

For the patient care competences, cluster 12 "consultation and assessment" (competences 43–45), the scores of hospital and community pharmacists were similar except for competence 43 "medical laboratory tests" where hospital pharmacists scored higher. There were six comments on cluster 12, with two on sectoral concerns. Four comments considered that "performing" laboratory tests is not important, whereas interpreting them is: *"Perform tests? I don't think that's relevant with regard to most laboratory tests. Interpretation is of course very important"*.

3.7. Cluster 13. Patient Care Competences: Need for Drug Treatment

For the patient care competences of cluster 13 "need for drug treatment" (competences 46–49), the scores of hospital and community pharmacists were similar. There were six comments on cluster 13. Five comments were on the issue of prescribing, e.g.: *"Pharmacists are not allowed to prescribe medicines as they do not know the patient's clinical background, and drug history"*; *"I think that prescribing would be important—unfortunately a theoretical concern at the moment"*; *"This would depend on the chosen career path following the pharmacy degree. I do not feel it appropriate for a newly qualified pharmacist to prescribe medication due to the lack of clinical experience unless the degree course is significantly extended and leads to specialist qualifications with significant clinical experience similar to doctor's training"*; and *"All pharmacists need to advise doctors but not essential to be able to prescribe."*

3.8. Cluster 14. Patient Care Competences: Drug Interactions

For the patient care competences of cluster 14 "drug interactions" (competences 50–52), the scores of hospital and community pharmacists were similar. There was one comment on cluster 14: *"This should be the expertise of the pharmacist."*

3.9. Cluster 15. Patient Care Competences: Provision of Drug Product

For the patient care competences cluster 15, "provision of drug product" (competences 53–57), the scores of hospital pharmacists were higher for competence 53 "pharmacodynamics and pharmacokinetics" and for competence 57 "ability to manufacture products." Concerning the latter there was a comment that *"Not sure how most pharmacists would be able to manufacture? Need for license etc."* It is to be noted that this is another example of possible confusion in that it could be argued that competence 57 belongs in the industrial pharmacy cluster 11.

3.10. Cluster 16. Patient Care Competences: Patient Education

For the patient care competences of cluster 16, "patient education" (competences 58–60), the scores of hospital pharmacists were lower than those of community pharmacies. There were no comments on this cluster.

3.11. Cluster 17. Patient Care Competences: Provision of Information and Service

For the patient care competences cluster 17, "provision of information and service" (competences 61–63), the scores of hospital and community pharmacists were similar except for competence 63 "non-prescription medicines" where the score of hospital pharmacists (78.9) whilst high, was substantially lower than that of community pharmacists (94.0). There were no comments on this cluster.

3.12. Cluster 18. Patient Care Competences: Monitoring of Drug Therapy

For the patient care competences in cluster 18, "monitoring of drug therapy" (competences 64–66), the scores of hospital pharmacists were similar to those of community pharmacies. There was one comment on this cluster: *"I am not sure that pharmacists know current clinical guidelines. If medicine is prescribed we give it to patient."*

3.13. Cluster 19. Patient Care Competences: Evaluation of Outcomes

For the patient care competences cluster 19, "evaluation of outcomes" (competences 67–68), the score of hospital pharmacists was higher regarding the cost effectiveness of treatment (competence 68). There were no comments on this cluster.

Overall the data suggest, firstly, that hospital and community pharmacists have similar ideas on the importance of various competences for practice. Secondly, it would appear that hospital pharmacists rank some of the competences in the context of their own specific activity suggesting that following on from this, certain competences are needed for certain specialisations. Continuing this argument further, after a ground-level competence-based course rooted in, for example, the PHAR-QA framework, certain competences may be necessary in terms of specialisation.

Similar arguments have been put forward for an "industrial pharmacy-oriented" master course given that practice in an industrial environment is very different from that in a community pharmacy environment. In the PHAR-QA survey, we included a cluster on industrial pharmacy; we chose not to include a cluster on hospital pharmacy as we considered that hospital and community practice have many similarities. This is backed up by the results. This does not exclude the fact that some topics such as radio-chemicals, preparation of drugs for specific pathologies, *etc.* are specifically part of hospital pharmacy practice (see later).

Hospital pharmacists taking part in this survey were not asked for their views on advanced-level competencies and there were few important differences between the hospital and community sectors. This is completely predicated on where these competencies are "located." Are they "registration" competencies (*i.e.*, applicable to all day 1 pharmacists—in other words a direct outcome of undergraduate/initial education) or are they "foundation" competencies (*i.e.*, related to scope of practice)? To gain further knowledge on this matter, a sub-analysis on the age of the respondents (in terms of two matched age groups) is presented in Figure 3. The duration of practical experience of specialists was considered as a main factor which could induce change and/or refinement of opinions concerning the basic competences required in pharmacy practice. Twenty years was considered as a threshold for change. Such a period is practically a generation. In previous generations, hospital pharmacy was more connected to industrial pharmacy with the preparation of, for example, perfusions for hospital wards and many semisolid formulations. In the same period, community pharmacy involved preparing formulations for short-term use requiring extensive knowledge of chemistry and pharmaceutical technology to avoid problems of stability, *etc.* It was expected that the disappearance of such competences would lead to differences in opinions between younger and older pharmacists. In this context, the duration of practice may be significant. However, as seen in Table 2, the number of responders with more than thirty years' experience was small (especially community pharmacists), so the effect of "experience" was estimated by effect of "age".

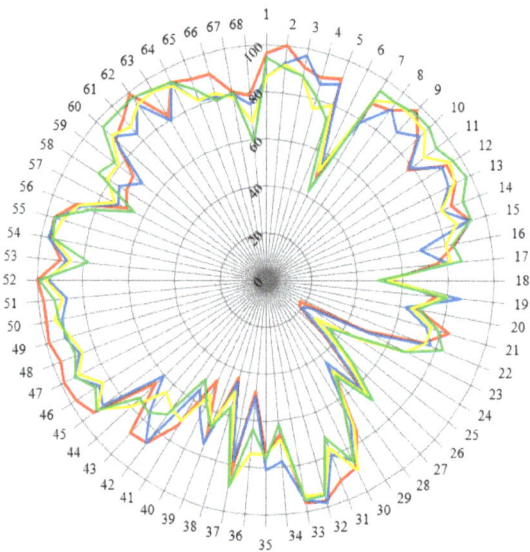

Figure 3. Scores (%) for rankings of competences for hospital and community pharmacists separated into two matched age groups. Hospital pharmacists: < 40 years old: red (*n* = 85), > 40 years old: blue (*n* = 110) Community pharmacists: < 40 years old: yellow (*n* = 148), > 40 years old: green (*n* = 67).

Figure 3 shows that the group "< 40 years old hospital pharmacists" is somewhat different for many competences especially those in the area of patient care competences. Significantly, there does not appear to be a clear difference between "registration" and "foundation" competences as there are more clear differences between this group and the group of older hospital pharmacists and between this group and age-matched community pharmacists This data would argue for an interaction between age and occupation.

A final consideration concerns the actual value of ranking competencies. One argument used by regulators of health professionals is that registered practitioners are either competent to perform or not. Ranking will imply degrees of competence, and in the eyes of regulators, degrees of patient safety. Furthermore, we can add a cautionary note that statistical difference does not imply an important difference when it comes to difference in a rank order; one example of this is competency 8, "demonstrate a professional approach to tasks and human relations" (90.1% for hospital *versus* 94.5% for community pharmacists), that shows a statistical difference, but represents, independently, a fundamental requirement of scope of practice, wherever you work.

4. Conclusions

In general, the agreement on the importance of competencies between different sectors of pharmaceutical activities is high. There was a large consensus between hospital and community pharmacists concerning "patient care", although the patients are not the same for the two groups. This is shown by the better score for clinical tests given by hospital pharmacists and the greater score given by community pharmacists to prescription drug competences. Other differences can be detected between community and hospital pharmacists. The higher focus of hospital pharmacists on knowledge of the different areas of science as well as on laboratory tests reflects the need of a hospital pharmacy specialisation as supported by the EAHP [14]. The difference is also visible in the field of drug production. This is a necessary competence in hospitals with requests for drugs for rare diseases, paediatric and oncologic drugs. Hospital pharmacists score entrepreneurship lower but cost-effectiveness higher than community pharmacists. This reflects the reality of pharmacy practice where community pharmacists have to act as entrepreneur and hospital pharmacists manage drug budgets. Some results for hospital pharmacists are surprising e.g., the lower score for human relations and patient education. This is probably the consequence of insufficient patient/pharmacist contact in ward rounds in a hospital, and needs some improvement.

This paper provides an innovative contribution to the literature on competence frameworks in pharmacy practice and education. To our knowledge this is the first time a competence framework developed by an academic team has been validated, using Delphi questionnaire methodology, by large populations of different pharmacy practitioners (community, hospital . . .). It is not the first competence framework for pharmacy practice to be proposed. Several previous frameworks [19,20] have been proposed but these were essentially the results of proposals by a panel of experts without subsequent validation by large numbers of pharmacy practitioners.

Our approach is based on that of the MEDINE group [18] who validated their proposal via a questionnaire sent out to European medical doctors and students. Results were similar to the ones presented here in that the medical community gave high ranking to competences related to general practice (carry out a consultation with a patient, assess clinical presentations, order investigations, make differential diagnoses, and negotiate a management plan, *etc.*). As in our study, the rankings of research topics were low (ability to design research experiments, ability to carry out practical laboratory research procedures, ability to analyse and disseminate experimental results [30], although a second study MEDINE2 suggested that stakeholders considered that "learning outcomes related both to "using research" and "doing research" should be core components of medical curricula" [18]. In contrast to our study, MEDINE looked only at the primary medical degree and did not investigate specialisation.

This paper also represents a first attempt to analyse ranking of competences for community and hospital pharmacy practice and, on the basis of this, to answer the questions: what is a community pharmacist? And what is a hospital pharmacist? Others have considered these questions. In a recent study to determine the use and relevance of the "National Competency Standards Framework for Pharmacists in Australia," it was found that students, interns and practising pharmacists had poor familiarity and use of the framework [31]. In a study in Thailand, 574 pharmacy practitioners and faculty members ranked pharmacy competency standards. The highest-ranked domain was Domain 1 "Practice Pharmacy within Laws, Professional Standards, and Ethics"; the second and third being

Domain 4 "Provide pharmaceutical care" and Domain 3 "Communicate and disseminate knowledge effectively" [32]. Such results are similar to those obtained here.

Other studies have given results different from those in this paper. The Elvey *et al.* [33] study "Who do you Think You Are? Pharmacists' Perceptions of Their Professional Identity," a panel of professional pharmacists (*n* = 43, community, hospital, primary care) were asked to give their opinions on the professional identity of the pharmacist. Semi-structured interviews were carried out with questions such as "Describe a pharmacist in five words." It was interesting that the strongest professional identity to emerge was the "scientist"—but there was considerable overlap with other identities. A somewhat similar conclusion was drawn by Waterfield [34], who asked the question "Is pharmacy a knowledge-based profession?" and found that the importance of the place of science in pharmacy curricula and practice was stressed.

In FIP (2008) [35], for example, several statements have been made regarding the goals and job description of the hospital pharmacy practitioner: "The overarching goal of hospital pharmacists is to optimize patient outcomes through the judicious, safe, efficacious, appropriate, and cost effective use of medicines" and "the 'five rights' (the right patient, right medicine, right dose, right route, and right time)." These obviously fit in with the priorities found in this paper as do the conclusions of other think-tank approaches such as that of the Society of Hospital Pharmacists of Australia [36] on general hospital pharmacy practice, and of others on more specialised areas such as clinical research [37]. However, to our knowledge, this is the first paper surveying the opinions of a large number of hospital pharmacy practitioners on their ideas on competences for practice.

5. Perspectives

In the light of the rankings and comments, a revised version of the competence framework has been sent out for survey. This will be the basis of the proposal of a PHAR-QA competence framework for pharmacy practice.

The interesting results of the survey support the initiative of the development of a common training framework for a hospital pharmacy post-graduated specialisation as supported by EAHP. The perception of the importance of some specific fields is already shown by the answers of hospital pharmacists. A note of caution is that the conclusions will increasingly be at odds with policy development across EU and wider. Learning from the mistakes made by medical workforce planning, regulators and policy makers now recognise that foundation training (*i.e.*, 2–3 years post-registration) should become the norm (for all sectors) and that advanced "generalism" is a key priority (patient demographics, primary care-based services, *etc.*). In addition, apart from a few competencies discussed here (which are less about "competency" and more about functional tasks—compounding, *etc.*), these outcomes rather suggest a majority similarly in ranking between sectors. The FIP conclusion is that there is significant (both importance and statistical) similarity in foundation competencies [38–40].

Acknowledgments: With the support of the Lifelong Learning programme of the European Union: 527194-LLP-1-2012-1-BE-ERASMUS-EMCR. This project has been funded with support from the European Commission. This publication reflects the views only of the authors; the Commission cannot be held responsible for any use which may be made of the information contained therein.

Author Contributions: Jeffrey Atkinson designed, constructed, ran and analysed the survey and wrote the paper. Kristien De Paepe ran the PHAR-QA consortium. Constantin Mircioiu played a major role in the conception of the statistical analyses; Constantin Mircioiu and Roxana Sandulovici checked and recalculated all the data. Antonio Sánchez Pozo and Dimitrios Rekkas developed the questionnaire. Antonio Sánchez Pozo, Dimitrios Rekkas, Jouni Hirvonen, Borut Bozic, Annie Marcincal and Agnieska Skowron helped with distribution of the survey. Constantin Mircioiu and Ian Bates played a major part in the writing and revision of the manuscript. Antonio Sánchez Pozo, Daisy Volmer, Keith A. Wilson, Andries Koster, Richard Price, Dimitrios Rekkas, and Kristien De Paepe provided useful criticism and suggestions during revision of the manuscript. Roberto Frontini and Richard Price from EAHP provided comments from the perspective of hospital pharmacy practice. Ian Bates suggested many useful modifications to the manuscript concerning the analysis and interpretation of the data and other aspects. Chris van Schravendijk assured the contacts with MEDINE. EAHP assured the distribution of the survey to their members.

Conflicts of Interest: The authors declare no conflict of interest.

Appendix A

Annex. Ranking of competences by hospital and community pharmacists. (Seq.: sequential numbering (as in figures). Note that the numbering of the clusters of competences starts at 7 (*i.e.*, continuing from the six questions on the profile of respondents). Competences in bold are those showing a statistically significant difference in distribution of rankings between groups (chi-square, $p < 0.05$).

Table A1. Scores (%) for the 68 competences for pharmacy practice as ranked by community and hospital pharmacists.

Cluster	Seq.	Competence	Hospital Pharmacists	Community Pharmacists
Cluster 7. Personal competences: learning and knowledge.	1	Ability to identify learning needs and to learn independently (including continuous professional development (CPD)).	91.4	89.8
	2	**Analysis: ability to apply logic to problem solving, evaluating pros and cons and following up on the solution found.**	96.7	91.1
	3	Synthesis: capacity to gather and critically appraise relevant knowledge and to summarise the key points.	94.0	87.9
	4	**Capacity to evaluate scientific data in line with current scientific and technological knowledge.**	88.0	75.8
	5	**Ability to interpret preclinical and clinical evidence-based medical science and apply the knowledge to pharmaceutical practice.**	89.3	75.9
	6	Ability to design and conduct research using appropriate methodology.	50.3	40.2
	7	**Ability to maintain current knowledge of relevant legislation and codes of pharmacy practice.**	84.0	91.7
Cluster 8. Personal competences: values.	8	**Demonstrate a professional approach to tasks and human relations.**	90.1	94.5
	9	**Demonstrate the ability to maintain confidentiality.**	92.1	95.3
	10	Take full personal responsibility for patient care and other aspects of one's practice.	90.1	94.8
	11	**Inspire confidence in others through actions and advice.**	78.1	88.8
	12	**Demonstrate high ethical standards.**	92.1	95.2

Table A1. *Cont.*

Cluster	Seq.	Competence	Hospital Pharmacists	Community Pharmacists
Cluster 9. Personal competences: communication and organisational skills.	13	Effective communication skills (both orally and written).	91.3	94.8
	14	Effective use of information technology.	88.7	86.1
	15	Ability to work effectively as part of a team.	92.7	89.2
	16	Ability to identify and implement legal and professional requirements relating to employment (e.g., for pharmacy technicians) and to safety in the workplace.	77.2	81.0
	17	Ability to contribute to the learning and training of staff.	76.4	82.5
	18	Ability to design and manage the development processes in the production of medicines.	50.7	43.2
	19	Ability to identify and manage risk and quality of service issues.	78.5	79.2
	20	Ability to identify the need for new services.	63.5	64.5
	21	Ability to communicate in English and/or locally relevant languages.	78.9	74.1
	22	Ability to evaluate issues related to quality of service.	74.3	77.9
	23	**Ability to negotiate, understand a business environment and develop entrepreneurship.**	**47.6**	**64.1**
Cluster 10. Personal competences: knowledge of different areas of the science of medicines.	24	**Plant and animal biology.**	**16.8**	**39.3**
	25	Physics.	16.8	21.7
	26	General and inorganic chemistry.	33.8	43.9
	27	Organic and medicinal/pharmaceutical chemistry.	61.6	66.0
	28	Analytical chemistry.	45.2	41.9
	29	General and applied biochemistry (medicinal and clinical).	72.8	68.8
	30	Anatomy and physiology; medical terminology.	87.8	88.7
	31	**Microbiology.**	**86.4**	**72.2**
	32	Pharmacology including pharmacokinetics.	98.0	94.7
	33	Pharmacotherapy and pharmaco-epidemiology.	95.9	94.3
	34	Pharmaceutical technology including analyses of medicinal products.	70.1	62.0
	35	Toxicology.	77.4	74.0
	36	**Pharmacognosy.**	**45.5**	**66.5**
	37	Legislation and professional ethics.	81.6	89.5

Table A1. *Cont.*

Cluster	Seq.	Competence	Hospital Pharmacists	Community Pharmacists
Cluster 11. Personal competences: understanding of industrial pharmacy.	38	Current knowledge of design, synthesis, isolation, characterisation and biological evaluation of active substances.	40.7	41.7
	39	**Current knowledge of good manufacturing practice (GMP) and of good laboratory practice (GLP).**	71.9	59.4
	40	**Current knowledge of European directives on qualified persons (QPs).**	52.2	43.7
	41	**Current knowledge of drug registration, licensing and marketing.**	64.0	55.7
	42	**Current knowledge of good clinical practice (GCP).**	86.4	64.5
Cluster 12. Patient care competences: patient consultation and assessment.	43	**Ability to perform and interpret medical laboratory tests.**	81.4	65.5
	44	Ability to perform appropriate diagnostic or physiological tests to inform clinical decision making e.g., measurement of blood pressure.	60.8	73.6
	45	Ability to recognise when referral to another member of the healthcare team is needed because a potential clinical problem is identified (pharmaceutical, medical, psychological or social).	91.8	91.7
Cluster 13. Patient care competences: need for drug treatment.	46	Retrieval and interpretation of relevant information on the patient's clinical background.	92.3	84.0
	47	Retrieval and interpretation of an accurate and comprehensive drug history if and when required.	95.8	91.5
	48	Identification of non-adherence and implementation of appropriate patient intervention.	92.2	86.8
	49	Ability to advise to physicians and—in some cases—prescribe medication.	93.6	87.6
Cluster 14. Patient care competences: drug interactions.	50	Identification, understanding and prioritisation of drug-drug interactions at a molecular level (e.g., use of codeine with paracetamol).	94.5	91.6
	51	Identification, understanding, and prioritisation of drug-patient interactions, including those that preclude or require the use of a specific drug (e.g., trastuzumab for treatment of breast cancer in women with HER2 overexpression).	93.1	89.7
	52	Identification, understanding, and prioritisation of drug-disease interactions (e.g., NSAIDs in heart failure).	97.9	96.6

Table A1. *Cont.*

Cluster	Seq.	Competence	Hospital Pharmacists	Community Pharmacists
Cluster 15. Patient care competences: provision of drug product.	53	**Familiarity with the bio-pharmaceutical, pharmacodynamic and pharmacokinetic activity of a substance in the body.**	88.8	81.2
	54	Supply of appropriate medicines taking into account dose, correct formulation, concentration, administration route and timing.	96.5	94.9
	55	Critical evaluation of the prescription to ensure that it is clinically appropriate and legal.	95.8	94.0
	56	Familiarity with the supply chain of medicines and the ability to ensure timely flow of drug products to the patient.	87.4	84.6
	57	**Ability to manufacture medicinal products that are not commercially available.**	67.6	60.5
Cluster 16. Patient care competences: patient education.	58	**Promotion of public health in collaboration with other actors in the healthcare system.**	72.2	82.6
	59	**Provision of appropriate lifestyle advice on smoking, obesity, etc.**	68.8	80.9
	60	**Provision of appropriate advice on resistance to antibiotics and similar public health issues.**	88.9	93.1
Cluster 17. Patient care competences: provision of information and service.	61	Ability to use effective consultations to identify the patient's need for information.	88.7	90.9
	62	Provision of accurate and appropriate information on prescription medicines.	96.5	94.4
	63	**Provision of informed support for patients in selection and use of non-prescription medicines for minor ailments (e.g., cough remedies ...).**	78.9	94.0
Cluster 18. Patient care competences: monitoring of drug therapy.	64	Identification and prioritisation of problems in the management of medicines in a timely manner and with sufficient efficacy to ensure patient safety.	93.0	93.0
	65	Ability to monitor and report to all concerned in a timely manner, and in accordance with current regulatory guidelines on Good Pharmacovigilance Practices (GVPs), Adverse Drug Events and Reactions (ADEs and ADRs).	85.9	83.4
	66	Undertaking of a critical evaluation of prescribed medicines to confirm that current clinical guidelines are appropriately applied.	86.3	80.6
Cluster 19. Patient care competences: evaluation of outcomes.	67	Assessment of outcomes on the monitoring of patient care and follow-up interventions.	80.3	79.0
	68	**Evaluation of cost effectiveness of treatment.**	76.6	61.2

The use of bold text designates competences where ranking frequencies showed a statistically significant difference using the chi-squared test ($p > 0.05$).

References

1. Search on "Web of Science". Available online: https://login.webofknowledge.com/error/Error? PathInfo=%2F&Alias=WOK5&Domain=.webofknowledge.com&Src=IP&RouterURL=https%3A%2F%2F www.webofknowledge.com%2F&Error=IPError (accessed on 20 May 2016).
2. The PHAR-QA: Quality Assurance in European Pharmacy Education and Training, Mission Statement. Available online: http://www.phar-qa.eu/mission-statement/ (accessed on 20 May 2016).
3. Directive 2004/38/EC of the European Parliament and of the Council of 29 April 2004 on the Right of Citizens of the Union and Their Family Members to Move and Reside Freely within the Territory of the Member States. Available online: http://eur-lex.europa.eu/legal-content/EN/TXT/PDF/?uri=CELEX: 32004L0038&from=FR (accessed on 20 May 2016).
4. The Bologna Process and the European Higher Education Area. Available online: http://ec.europa.eu/ education/policy/higher-education/bologna-process_en.htm (accessed on 20 May 2016).
5. Atkinson, J.; Rombaut, B. The 2011 PHARMINE report on pharmacy and pharmacy education in the European Union. *Pharm. Pract. (Internet)* **2011**, *9*, 169–187. [CrossRef]
6. The International Pharmaceutical Federation (FIP). Global Pharmacy Workforce Report. 2012. Available online: http://www.fip.org/humanresources (accessed on 20 May 2016).
7. Ordre des Pharmaciens, France, Eléments Démographiques. Les Pharmaciens, Panorama au 1er Janvier 2014. Available online: http://www.ordre.pharmacien.fr/Communications/Elements-demographiques/ Les-pharmaciens-Panorama-au-1er-janvier-2015 (accessed on 20 May 2016).
8. ABDA, Bundesvereinigung Deutscher Apotheker Verbände. Jahresbericht 13/14. Available online: http://www.abda.de/service/publikationen/jahresbericht/ (accessed on 20 May 2016).
9. Consejo General de Colegios Oficiales de Farmacéuticos. Available online: http://www.portalfarma.com/ Paginas/default.aspx (accessed on 20 May 2016).
10. General Pharmaceutical Council (GPhC). Registrant Survey 2013. Available online: https://www. pharmacyregulation.org/sites/default/files/gphc_all_registrant_survey_2013_-_infographics.pdf (accessed on 20 May 2016).
11. The European Union. The Council Directive of 16 September 1985 Concerning the Coordination of Provisions Laid down by Law, Regulation or Administrative Action in Respect of Certain Activities in the Field of Pharmacy. Available online: http://eur-lex.europa.eu/legal-content/EN/TXT/PDF/?uri=CELEX: 31985L0432&from=EN (accessed on 20 May 2016).
12. The European Union. The EU directive 2013/55/EU on the Recognition of Professional Qualifications, Article 49a. Available online: http://eur-lex.europa.eu/legal-content/EN/TXT/?uri=CELEX:02005L0036-20140117 (accessed on 20 May 2016).
13. The European Common Training Framework "CTF". Available online: http://www.eahp.eu/press-room/ european-parliament-improves-professional-qualification-rules (accessed on 20 May 2016).
14. The Common Training Framework in Hospital Pharmacy. Available online: http://www.hospitalpharmacy. eu (accessed on 20 May 2016).
15. Minghetti, P.; Pantano, D.; Grazia, C.; Gennari, M.; Casiraghi, A. Regulatory framework of pharmaceutical compounding and actual developments of legislation in Europe. *Health Policy* **2014**, *117*, 328–333. [CrossRef] [PubMed]
16. The PHAR-QA project: Quality Assurance in European Pharmacy Education and Training. Work Package 2 "Implementation". Available online: http://www.phar-qa.eu/wp-content/uploads/2014/05/PHAR_ QA_WP2_Implementation.pdf (accessed on 20 May 2016).
17. The PHARMINE "Pharmacy education in Europe" Project, Final Reports. Available online: http://www. pharmine.org/pharmine/final-report/ (accessed on 20 May 2016).
18. Marz, R.; Dekker, F.W.; van Schravendijk, C.; O'Flynn, S.; Ross, M.T. Tuning research competences for Bologna three cycles in medicine: Report of a MEDINE2 European consensus survey. *Perspect. Med. Educ.* **2013**, *2*, 181–195. [CrossRef] [PubMed]
19. CoDEG (Competency Development and Evaluation Group). General Level Practice. Available online: http://www.codeg.org/frameworks/general-level-practice/ (accessed on 20 May 2016).

20. Stupans, I.; McAllister, S.; Clifford, R.; Hughes, J.; Krass, I.; March, G.; Owen, S.; Woulfeg, J. Nationwide collaborative development of learning outcomes and exemplar standards for Australian pharmacy programmes. *Int. J. Pharm. Pract.* **2015**, *23*, 283–291. [CrossRef] [PubMed]

21. The PHAR-QA European Delphi Round 1 Survey. Available online: http://www.phar-qa.eu/wp-content/uploads/2015/03/PHAR_QA_EU_network_Delphi_1_201503.pdf (accessed on 20 May 2016).

22. Atkinson, J.; de Paepe, K.; Sánchez Pozo, A.; Rekkas, D.; Volmer, D.; Hirvonen, J.; Bozic, B.; Skowron, A.; Mircioiu, C.; Marcincal, A.; *et al.* The PHAR-QA Project: Competency Framework for Pharmacy Practice—First Steps, the Results of the European Network Delphi Round 1. *Pharmacy* **2015**, *3*, 307–329. [CrossRef]

23. Leik, R.K. A measure of ordinal consensus. In *The Pacific Sociological Review*; University of California Press: Oakland, CA, USA, 1966; Volume 9, pp. 85–90.

24. GraphPad Software, Inc. GraphPad Statistical Pack. Available online: http://www.graphpad.com/ (accessed on 20 May 2016).

25. Qualitative Data Systems Analysis. Qualitative Data Analysis Software (QSR). Available online: http://www.qsrinternational.com/products_nvivo.aspx (accessed on 20 May 2016).

26. Smith, A.E.; Humphreys, M.S. Evaluation of unsupervised semantic mapping of natural language with Leximancer concept mapping. *Behav. Res. Methods.* **2006**, *38*, 262–279. [CrossRef] [PubMed]

27. Comunicat al Comisiei Comisiei Nationale de Bioetica a Medicamentului si a Dispozitivelor Medicale. Available online: http://www.adsm.ro/ro (accessed on 20 May 2016).

28. Grabowski, H. The Evolution of the Pharmaceutical Industry over the Past 50 Years: A Personal Reflection. *Int. J. Econ. Bus.* **2011**, *18*, 161–176. [CrossRef]

29. McElhiney, L.F. Compounding for children: The compounding pharmacist. Paediatric formulations: A roadmap. *AAPS Adv. Pharm. Sci. Ser.* **2014**, *11*, 329–334.

30. The Tuning Network. MEDINE—Medicine (2004–2007 & 2009–2013). Available online: http://tuningacademy.org/medine-medicine/?lang=en (accessed on 20 May 2016).

31. Nash, R.E.; Chalmers, L.; Stupans, I.; Brown, N. Knowledge, use and perceived relevance of a profession's Competency Standards; implications for Pharmacy Education. *Int. J. Pharm. Pract.* **2016**. [CrossRef] [PubMed]

32. Maitreemit, P.; Pongcharoensuk, P.; Kapol, N.; Armstrong, E.P. Pharmacist Perceptions of New Competency Standards. *Pharm. Pract.* **2008**, *6*, 113–120. [CrossRef]

33. Elvey, R.; Hassell, K.; Hall, K. Who do you Think You Are? Pharmacists' Perceptions of Their Professional Identity. *Int. J. Pharm. Pract.* **2013**, *21*, 322–332. [CrossRef] [PubMed]

34. Waterfield, J. Is pharmacy a knowledge-based profession? *Am. J. Pharm. Educ.* **2010**, *74*, 1–6. [CrossRef]

35. FIP Global Conference on the Future of Hospital Pharmacy (2008). Available online: https://www.fip.org/files/fip/HPS/Basel2008/translations/BaselStatementsFrench.pdf (accessed on 20 May 2016).

36. Dooley, M.; Dowling, H.; Eaton, V.; Kirsa, S.; Maunsell, T.; Roberts, A.; Ryan, M. Identifying priorities for the pharmacy profession: The SHPA 2014 Future Summit. *J. Pharm. Pract. Res.* **2015**, *45*, 76–80. [CrossRef]

37. Poloyac, S.M.; Empey, K.M.; Rohan, L.C.; Skledar, S.J.; Empey, P.E.; Nolin, T.D.; Bies, R.R.; Gibbs, R.B.; Folan, M.; Kroboth, P.D. Instructional design and assessment. Core Competencies for Research Training in the Clinical Pharmaceutical Sciences. *Am. J. Pharm. Educ.* **2011**. [CrossRef]

38. Meštrovića, A.; Staničić, Z.; Ortner Hadžiabdić, M.; Mucalo, I.; Bates, I.; Duggan, C.; Carter, S.; Bruno, A. Community pharmacists' competency evaluation and education using the general level framework in Croatia. *Am. J. Pharm. Educ.* **2011**, *75*, 36. [CrossRef]

39. Rutter, V.; Wong, C.; Coombes, I.; Cardiff, L.; Duggan, C.; Yee, M.-L.; Lim, K.W.; Bates, I. Use of a General Level Framework to Facilitate Performance Improvement in Hospital Pharmacists in Singapore. *Am. J. Pharm. Educ.* **2012**. [CrossRef] [PubMed]

40. Coombes, I.; Avent, M.; Cardiff, L.; Bettenay, K.; Coombes, J.; Whitfield, K.; Stokes, J.; Davies, G.; Bates, I. Improvement in Pharmacist's Performance Facilitated by an Adapted Competency-Based General Level Framework. *J. Pharm. Pract. Res.* **2010**, *40*, 111–118. [CrossRef]

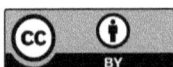

pharmacy

MDPI

Article

A Study on How Industrial Pharmacists Rank Competences for Pharmacy Practice: A Case for Industrial Pharmacy Specialization

Jeffrey Atkinson [1,*], Kristien De Paepe [2], Antonio Sánchez Pozo [3], Dimitrios Rekkas [4], Daisy Volmer [5], Jouni Hirvonen [6], Borut Bozic [7], Agnieska Skowron [8], Constantin Mircioiu [9], Annie Marcincal [10], Andries Koster [11], Keith Wilson [12] and Chris van Schravendijk [13]

[1] Pharmacolor Consultants Nancy, 12 rue de Versigny, Villers 54600, France
[2] Pharmacy Faculty, Vrije Universiteit Brussel, Laarbeeklaan 103, Brussels 1090, Belgium; kdepaepe@vub.ac.be
[3] Faculty of Pharmacy, University of Granada (UGR), Campus Universitario de la Cartuja s/n, Granada 18701, Spain; sanchezp@ugr.es
[4] School of Pharmacy, National and Kapodistrian University Athens, Panepistimiou 30, Athens 10679, Greece; rekkas@pharm.uoa.gr
[5] Pharmacy Faculty, University of Tartu, Nooruse 1, Tartu 50411, Estonia; daisy.volmer@ut.ee
[6] Pharmacy Faculty, University of Helsinki, Yliopistonkatu 4, P.O. Box 33-4, Helsinki 00014, Finland; jouni.hirvonen@helsinki.fi
[7] Faculty of Pharmacy, University of Ljubljana, Askerceva cesta 7, Ljubljana 1000, Slovenia; Borut.Bozic@ffa.uni-lj.si
[8] Pharmacy Faculty, Jagiellonian University, UL, Golebia 24, Krakow 31-007, Poland; askowron@cm-uj.krakow.pl
[9] Pharmacy Faculty, University of Medicine and Pharmacy "Carol Davila" Bucharest, Dionisie Lupu 37, Bucharest 020021, Romania; constantin.mircioiu@yahoo.com
[10] European Association of Faculties of Pharmacy, Faculty of Pharmacy, Université de Lille 2 , Lille 59000, France; annie.marcincal@pharma.univ-lille2.fr
[11] European Association of Faculties of Pharmacy, Department of Pharmaceutical Sciences, Utrecht University, PO Box 80082, Utrecht 3508 TB, The Netherlands; A.S.Koster@uu.nl
[12] Applied Health Research Unit, School of Life and Health Sciences, Aston University, Birmingham B4 7ET, UK; k.a.wilson@aston.ac.uk
[13] Medical Faculty, Vrije Universiteit Brussel, Laarbeeklaan 103, Brussels 1090, Belgium; chrisvs@vub.ac.be
* Correspondence: jeffrey.atkinson@univ-lorraine.fr; Tel./Fax: +33-383-27-37-03

Academic Editor: Yvonne Perrie
Received: 25 November 2015; Accepted: 22 January 2016; Published: 6 February 2016

Abstract: This paper looks at the way in which industrial pharmacists rank the fundamental competences for pharmacy practice. European industrial pharmacists ($n = 135$) ranked 68 competences for practice, arranged into 13 clusters of two types (personal and patient care). Results show that, compared to community pharmacists ($n = 258$), industrial pharmacists rank competences centering on research, development and production of drugs higher, and those centering on patient care lower. Competences centering on values, communication skills, *etc.* were ranked similarly by the two groups of pharmacists. These results are discussed in the light of the existence or not of an "industrial pharmacy" specialization.

Keywords: education; specialization; practice

---

1. Introduction

Graduates with a pharmacy degree are employed in a variety of positions, the most important (in terms of numbers) being community, hospital and industrial pharmacy. The discussion on whether these three domains require specific skills with a specific education has long been contentious. Industrial pharmacy as a university discipline is recognized by some European pharmacy departments. The PHARMINE study (*Pharmacy Education in Europe*) reported that pharmacy departments in 10/31 European countries give elective pre-graduate courses in industrial pharmacy, and 11/31 departments give post-graduate industrial pharmacy courses [1]. Most of the graduates from such courses go on to to work in an industrial setting. The PHARMINE study reported that a substantial number (37,308) of European pharmacists (6% of the industrial workforce) work in the pharmaceutical industry [2]; this is similar to the worldwide figure of 10% given by the International Pharmaceutical Federation [3].

In some European countries the status of the industrial pharmacist is officially recognized. In France, the profession of "industrial pharmacist" is defined by national law and the statutes of the pharmacy professional body [4]. On the global European level, this is not the case. In the European Union (EU), the 1985 EU directive on the profession of pharmacy [5], and the 2013 update [6], do not recognize any specialization in pharmacy (although these are recognized in medicine).

There is a second EU directive that is relevant in this case, however, and that is the EU directive on qualified persons working in the pharmaceutical industry [7]. In some EU member states, such as Germany [8], only those with a pharmacy degree meet the requirements set down in the qualified persons directive.

It appears, therefore, that the argument is equivocal for the existence of a specialized pharmacy job description of "industrial pharmacist" (*i.e.*, a pharmacist working in industry) that is different from that of other specialties such as community pharmacy. This paper looks at one aspect of this discussion: whether industrial pharmacists rank competences for practice differently than do community pharmacists. It is possible that pharmacists working within such specialties view the pharmacy profession differently. Within this context we investigated, therefore, whether the ranking by industrial pharmacists of competences for practice is different from that of community pharmacists.

In the PHAR-QA ("*Quality Assurance in European PHARmacy Education and Training*") project [9], we asked community and industrial pharmacists to rank competences for pharmacy practice. This paper describes the similarities and differences between the ways in which European industrial and community pharmacists respectively rank competences for pharmacy practice.

2. Experimental Section

Ranking data on competences for practice were obtained using the PHAR-QA *surveymonkey* [10] questionnaire that was available online from 14 February 2014 to 1 November 2014, *i.e.*, 8.5 months [11]. Respondents came from 36/49 countries of the European Higher Education Area [12].

The first six questions were on the profile of the respondent (duration of practice, country of residence, current occupation (industrial, community … pharmacist)). There was also a question on the job title. This allowed a subdivision of industrial pharmacists according to their experience/activity: regulatory affairs, research and development, *etc.* A similar subdivision of the activities of community pharmacists was not possible, as all respondents in this group were involved in some form of dispensation to patients.

Questions 7 through 19 asked about 13 clusters of 68 competences (see Appendix A). Questions in clusters 7 to 11 were concerned with personal competences, and in clusters 12 to 19 with patient care competences.

Respondents were asked to rank the proposals for competences on a 4-point Likert scale:

(1) Not important = Can be ignored;
(2) Quite important =Valuable but not obligatory;
(3) Very important = Obligatory, with exceptions depending upon field of pharmacy practice;
(4) Essential = Obligatory.

There was also a "cannot rank" possibility as well as that of leaving the answer blank.
Results are presented in the form of "scores" calculated as follows:

Ranking score = (frequency rank 3 + frequency rank 4) as % of total frequency, which represents the percentage of respondents that considered a given competence as "obligatory".

This calculation is based on a similar calculation made by the MEDINE consortium that studied the ranking of competences for medical practice [13]. Such scores are used for descriptive purposes only, and no conclusions on statistical differences amongst groups are based on scores.

Leik ordinal consensus [14] was calculated as an indication of the dispersion of the data using an Excel spreadsheet. The original Leik paper cited previously gives an explicit mathematical example of the calculation of ordinal consensus. Responses for consensus were arbitrarily classified as: < 0.2 poor, 0.21–0.4 fair, 0.41–0.6 moderate, 0.61–0.8 substantial, > 0.81 good, according to the scale used in MEDINE study.

The statistical significance of differences between rankings of competences or between rankings by different categories of respondents was tested by the chi-square test (confidence level 95%). Statistical tests were performed using GraphPad software [15].

Results are presented at 2 levels: that of the 13 clusters and that of the 68 competences.

Respondents could also add their comments on the different clusters. An attempt was made to analyze comments using the NVivo10 program [16] for the semi-quantitative analysis of unstructured data. It was found that the numbers involved were too small to draw significant conclusions.

3. Results and Discussion

The distribution by duration of practice of the groups is given in Table 1.

Table 1. Distribution of duration of practice (years) in industrial and community pharmacist responders. *n*: number in each category.

Respondents	< 5	6–10	11–20	21–40	Blank	Total
Industrial pharmacists (*n*)	26	31	28	23	27	135
Community pharmacists (*n*)	50	51	41	56	60	258

Most respondents had less than 20 years of experience, thus in both cases a relatively "young" population was involved. This may be due to the higher motivation of a younger population to reply to a questionnaire.

Respondents came from 36 European countries. Nineteen countries provided 5 or more respondents to one or both groups; they were: Belgium, Croatia, Czech Republic, Estonia, Finland, Germany, Greece, Hungary, Ireland, Italy, Macedonia, Montenegro, Norway, Romania, Slovenia, Spain, Switzerland, The Netherlands, and the United Kingdom.

The numbers of industrial pharmacy respondents arranged according to experience/activity are given in Table 2.

Table 2. Numbers of industrial pharmacy respondents subdivided according to experience/activity.

Experience/Activity	Number
Management	24
Regulatory affairs	23
Research and development	18
Quality assurance/compliance	16
Pharmaceutical technology	10
Clinical/medical affairs	8
Pharmacovigilance	5
Qualified person	5
Marketing and sales	5
Research student/Ph.D.	1
"Industrial pharmacist" or "pharmacist"	8
Blank	12

Table 2 shows that, while some respondents work in a typically "pharmaceutical" environment (such as regulatory affairs and pharmaceutical technology), many others work in more "generic" environments (such as management and quality assurance). If we consider that industrial surroundings correspond to 4 groups/stages, namely (1) research and development; (2) production; (3) analyses and quality assurance; and (4) marketing and sales, it appears that not all pharmacists employed in marketing and sales feel that they are industrial pharmacists. Indeed, marketing and sales representatives of "big pharma" are sometimes very far from classical industrial surroundings, even though they are employed in industry.

Table 3 shows the overall distribution of rankings by industrial and community pharmacists.

Table 3. Overall distribution (over 13 clusters of 68 competences) of rankings by industrial and community pharmacists.

Ranking	Industrial Pharmacists		Community Pharmacists	
Number of respondents	138		258	
Theoretical number of replies	9384 (= 138 × 68)		17,544 (= 258 × 68)	
Rank	Number	%	Number	%
4	2510	26.8	6643	37.9
3	3502	37.3	6002	34.2
2	1876	20.0	3076	17.5
1	432	4.6	608	3.5
Cannot rank + blanks	1064	11.3	1215	6.9
Score (%)	=((2510 + 3502)/8320) × 100 = 72.3		= ((6643 + 6002)/16,329) × 100 = 77.4	
Leik ordinal consensus	0.58		0.55	

Notes: Chi-square test on distribution of ranks for industrial *versus* community pharmacists: $p < 0.05$ (degrees of freedom = 3, ((4 ranks −1) × (2 groups −1)).

All but 7–11% of respondents were able to rank all competences. This suggests that the majority in both groups of respondents believed that they were sufficiently informed to reply to almost all the questions asked.

As judged from the Leik ordinal consensus values, dispersion was low. This suggests that both groups were relatively homogeneous and that subgroups with responses significantly different from the overall group do not exist. Similar values for ordinal consensus have been reported by the MEDINE consortium.

Overall ranking by industrial pharmacists was significantly lower (72%) than that by community pharmacists (77%). This raises the question of whether industrial pharmacists globally believed that the competence framework was less applicable; however, the global score was high with almost 3/4 of industrial pharmacists considering the competences "obligatory". The global lower score of industrial pharmacists was weighted by the low scores they gave to patient care competences (see later).

Figures 1 and 2 show the results for analysis by clusters. In Figure 1, the values for Leik ordinal consensus are shown.

Leik ordinal consensus was higher for industrial pharmacists in 10/13 clusters including cluster 11 that dealt with competences for industrial pharmacy.

Scores for personal competences (clusters 7 to 11) were similar in industrial and community pharmacists, except for cluster 11, dealing with industrial pharmacy, for which industrial pharmacists scored higher. Scores for clusters dealing with patient care competences (clusters 12 to 19) were lower for industrial pharmacists.

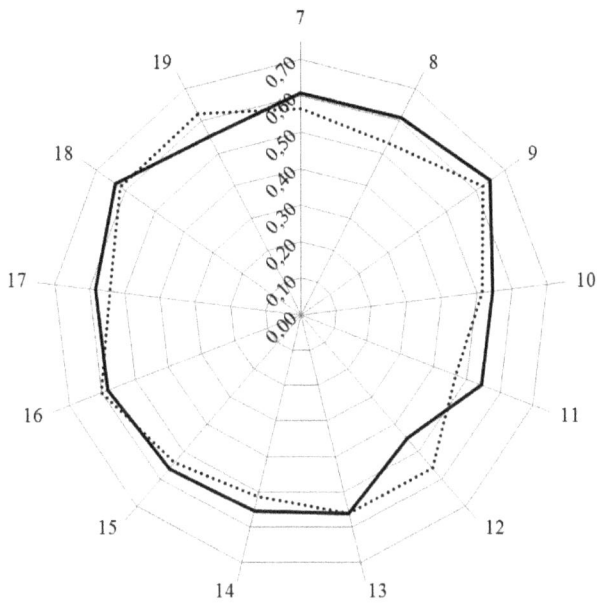

Figure 1. Leik ordinal consensus for rankings by clusters for industrial (solid line) and community (dotted line) pharmacists.

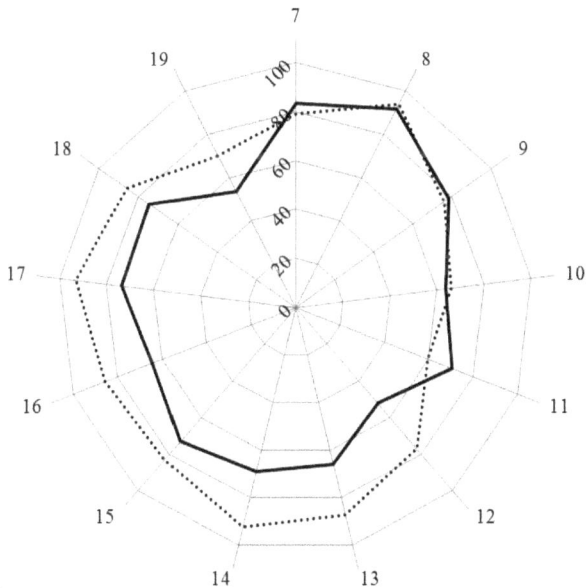

Figure 2. Scores (%) for rankings by clusters for industrial (solid line) and community (dotted line) pharmacists.

Figures 3 and 4 show the results for analysis by competences. In Figure 3, the values for Leik ordinal consensus are shown.

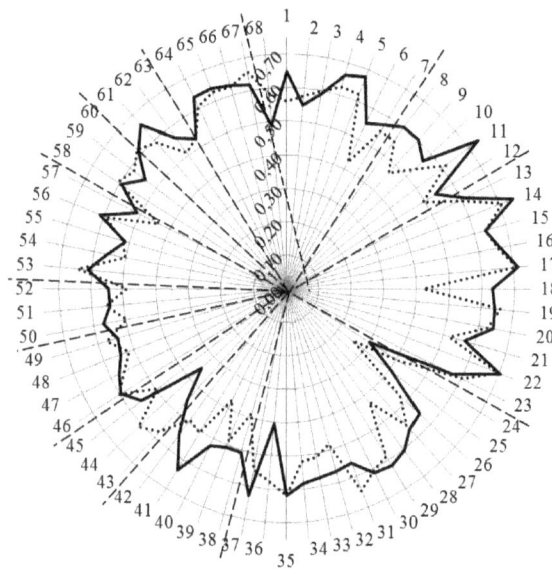

Figure 3. Leik ordinal consensus for rankings by competences for industrial (solid line) and community (dotted line) pharmacists. Dashed lines separate the different clusters of competences.

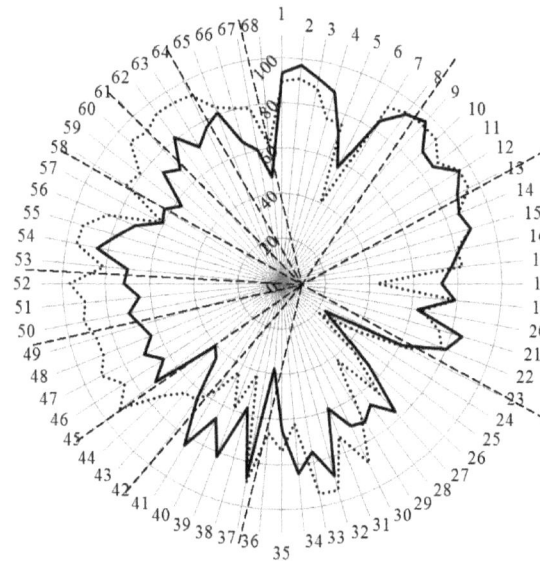

Figure 4. Scores (%) for rankings by competences for industrial (solid line) and community (dotted line) pharmacists. Dashed lines separate the different clusters of competences.

Overall, the ordinal consensus values were higher for industrial than for community pharmacists. This was especially true for competences 6 (research), 18 (development, production of medicines), 28 (analytical chemistry), 38 (design, synthesis, *etc.* of active substances), 40 (EU directive on qualified persons), and 41 (drug registration, licensing and marketing). For all these competences, the consensus for industrial pharmacists was higher than community pharmacists (Figure 4 and Appendix A). For competences 31 (microbiology) and 44 (diagnostic tests) the ordinal consensus for community pharmacists was higher than that for industrial pharmacists, as were the scores (Figure 4 and Appendix A).

Scores for the 68 competences are given in Figure 4 and the Appendix A.

This graph shows that competences on the right-hand side concerned with personal values, subject matters and industrial pharmacy were often ranked higher by industrial pharmacists. Competences on the left-hand side concerned with patient care were often ranked higher by community pharmacists. A proviso must be added here; through a comparison between Figure 4 with Figure 3, it is obvious that, for competences scoring low (e.g., 24 and 25), consensus was low. Thus, the low ranking was far from unanimous.

Going into more detail, Table 4 shows the competences for which industrial pharmacist ranked higher (upper) and for which community pharmacists ranked higher (lower).

Table 4. Competences ranked higher by industrial pharmacist (upper) and by community pharmacists (lower). (**a**) Industrial > community; (**b**) Community > industrial.

(**a**)

n	Competence
4	Capacity to evaluate scientific data in line with current scientific and technological knowledge
6	Ability to design and conduct research using appropriate methodology
18	Ability to design and manage the development processes in the production of medicines
25	Physics
28	Analytical chemistry
34	Pharmaceutical technology including analyses of medicinal products
38	Current knowledge of design, synthesis, isolation, characterization and biological evaluation of active substances
39	Current knowledge of good manufacturing practice (GMP) and of good laboratory practice (GLP)
40	Current knowledge of European directives on qualified persons (QPs)
41	Current knowledge of drug registration, licensing and marketing

(**b**)

n	Competence
24	Plant and animal biology
30	Anatomy and physiology; medical terminology
33	Pharmacotherapy and pharmaco-epidemiology
36	Pharmacognosy
43	Ability to perform and interpret medical laboratory tests
44	Ability to perform appropriate diagnostic or physiological tests to inform clinical decision making (e.g., measurement of blood pressure)
45	Ability to recognise when referral to another member of the healthcare team is needed because a potential clinical problem is identified (pharmaceutical, medical, psychological or social)
46	Retrieval and interpretation of relevant information on the patient's clinical background
47	Retrieval and interpretation of an accurate and comprehensive drug history if and when required
48	Identification of non-adherence and implementation of appropriate patient intervention
49	Ability to advise to physicians and, in some cases, prescribe medication
50	Identification, understanding and prioritization of drug-drug interactions at a molecular level (e.g., use of codeine with paracetamol)
51	Identification, understanding, and prioritization of drug-patient interactions, including those that preclude or require the use of a specific drug (e.g., trastuzumab for treatment of breast cancer in women with HER2 overexpression)
52	Identification, understanding, and prioritization of drug-disease interactions (e.g., NSAIDs in heart failure)
55	Critical evaluation of the prescription to ensure that it is clinically appropriate and legal
56	Familiarity with the supply chain of medicines and the ability to ensure timely flow of drug products to the patient

Table 4. *Cont.*

n	Competence
58	Promotion of public health in collaboration with other actors in the healthcare system
59	Provision of appropriate lifestyle advice on smoking, obesity, *etc.*
60	Provision of appropriate advice on resistance to antibiotics and similar public health issues
61	Ability to use effective consultations to identify the patient's need for information
62	Provision of accurate and appropriate information on prescription medicines
63	Provision of informed support for patients in selection and use of non-prescription medicines for minor ailments (e.g., cough remedies)
64	Identification and prioritization of problems in the management of medicines in a timely manner and with sufficient efficacy to ensure patient safety
66	Undertaking of a critical evaluation of prescribed medicines to confirm that current clinical guidelines are appropriately applied
67	Assessment of outcomes on the monitoring of patient care and follow-up interventions
68	Evaluation of cost effectiveness of treatment

The competences ranked higher by industrial pharmacists fall into three groups with, firstly, competences 4, 6 and 18 on evaluation of scientific data, research, and production of medicines. Scores for community pharmacists on 2 of these competences (6, 18) were less than 50%. The second group was concerned with the subject matters physics (25) 33%, analytical chemistry (28) 67%, and pharmaceutical technology (34) 84%. Subject matters were included because they figure in the EU directive on the sectoral profession of pharmacy. The authors recognize that they are not competences but part of the foundation of competences. Having said that, it should be noted that community pharmacists ranked these elements very low, with a score of 22% for physics and 42% for analytical chemistry. Thus, the general message that all the subject matters cited in the EU directive are essential for science-based pharmacy practice is not understood, as concerns subjects such as physics.

In the lower part of Table 4, the competences that are ranked higher by community pharmacists are shown. Four of these concern subject areas (24, 30, 33, and 36), but the majority concern patient care competences. For the latter community pharmacists scored significantly higher than industrial pharmacists for all but five competences. This is not to say that industrial pharmacists scored low for patient care competences, as almost all of their scores were between 60% and 80%. Thus, they do recognize the need for information relating to the pharmacist as a medicine specialist (see also comments below).

Overall, the observations in the previous paragraphs suggest that the two groups are often ranking in the context of their own specific activity and, following on from this, that certain competences are needed for certain specializations. Continuing this argument further, certain competences could thus be part of an "industrial pharmacy-oriented" degree course, and others part of a "community pharmacy-oriented" degree course (taking for example, those in Table 4). An alternative argument is that this is in favor of "amplifying" different clusters in different specializations within a single curriculum, rather than "separating" competences into different curricula for the two activities.

Comments were made by 15/138 (11%) of industrial pharmacist and 23/258 (9%) of community pharmacist respondents. Our initial objective was to evaluate whether comments were in line with scoring, but the low numbers of comments received did not permit a satisfactory analysis using semi-quantitative analysis of unstructured data (results not shown). Comments are reported here, therefore, in a "raw data" form.

Comments are grouped into areas in Table 5.

There were several comments on the English phraseology and the construction of the questions, and these have been taken into consideration in the production of the revised version of the questionnaire. Others pointed to the esoteric nature of certain competences and the recognition of specialization, be it industrial or community. Of interest also is the fact that industrial pharmacists recognized the necessity of all competences, including patient care competences, and the nature of the pharmacist as a "medicines specialist".

Table 5. Comments by industrial and community pharmacists.

Area	Typical Examples of Comments Made.	
	Industrial Pharmacist.	Community Pharmacist.
Understanding of the question	- I do not understand the question. - I have not spoken English for a long time. - One point only to each question. - Important to interpret but not necessarily done.	- The question is very convoluted. - The question is rather unclear.
Production of medicines.		We buy rather than produce them.
Information sources.		- I get all my information (on drugs) from reliable sources. - Pre-selection of new scientific information by official institutes.
Framework for community pharmacy practice.	- Being a pharmacist, you need basic information in all areas. - Although I work in industry, all these competences are needed. - The pharmacist is a medicines specialist. - Response depends on the area you are working in.	- All answers refer to daily work in a community pharmacy. - Answers relate to my working environment. - Pharmaceutical care is essential. - Some competences are for specialists. - Some competences are for hospital pharmacists.
Economics/business administration.	Cost effectiveness assessment is a specialist role.	- It is vital to have economics and business administration. - "Business environment," yes, but keep your eye on the health aspect. - Pharmacists follow recommendations of NICE not cost effectiveness.
No prescription.		- Pharmacists are not allowed to prescribe in my country. - Pharmacists are not physicians.
Healthcare team.		Pharmacists are responsible for their part of the job.
Subject areas.	- You need basic knowledge of all areas. - Pharmacognosy is no longer a required subject. - Radio-pharmacy would be useful.	We do not need analytical chemistry as we are not analyzing any more.
Industrial pharmacy/research.	- These apply to industrial pharmacists. - These competences are esoteric. - Preclinical issues are not part of my work experience.	- I have never worked in industry. - These competences are for industry and research.
Consultation/diagnosis.		- A pharmacist is not a doctor. - It is not uncommon that the pharmacist is the first person to whom the patient explains his symptoms. - We are not appropriately trained for this. - Commercial interests are involved.

Globally, the comments leave a subjective impression of backing up the scores, but, as explained in Section 2, no solid conclusions can be drawn.

4. Conclusions

Competences centering on values, communication skills, *etc.* were ranked similarly by the two groups of pharmacists (industrial and community). In other areas, such as (1) drug research, development and production, and (2) patient care, scores suggest that the groups appeared to be ranking in the context of their own specific activity. These results are discussed in the light of the existence of, or need for, an "industrial pharmacy" specialization based on a specific competence framework. The latter is provided by the PHAR-QA framework.

The pharmacists' perception of their profession is primarily determined within the context of their specific activities in their line of work. The split in opinion lies between "hard sciences" and "patient care." The truth is that the pharmacy service that best serves the population at large involves both. Pharmacy students seldom know in advance whether they will end up working as industrial or as community pharmacists. Taking this into account, one could argue that a pharmacist should receive a balanced education involving the two areas and then specialize in one of the two as his/her professional career advances, post-registration. On the other hand, if the degree of specialization necessary is so profound that it would be best to start it from the educational phase, the specialty-oriented program may be the better solution. The discussion on this dilemma continues.

5. Perspectives

In light of the rankings and comments, a revised version of the competence framework will be sent out for survey. This will be followed by the proposal of a PHAR-QA competence framework for pharmacy practice.

Future papers will deal with results for hospital pharmacists, and academics. These papers, as does the present paper, will deal with the implications of the results obtained, thus contributing to the ongoing debate on the perceptions of professional identity of a pharmacist [17], in this case, with contributions that are backed up by hard data.

Acknowledgments: With the support of the Lifelong Learning program of the European Union: 527194-LLP-1-2012-1-BE-ERASMUS-EMCR, this project has been funded with support from the European Commission. This publication reflects the views only of the author; the Commission cannot be held responsible for any use which may be made of the information contained therein. The authors thank Jane Nicholson of the European Industrial Pharmacists' Group (EIPG), Vivian Moffat of the European Federation of Pharmaceutical Industries and Associations (EFPIA), and Hans Linden of the European Federation for Pharmaceutical Sciences (EUFEPS) for distributing the PHAR-QA questionnaire to the members of their associations.

Author Contributions: Jeffrey Atkinson designed, constructed, ran and analyzed the survey and wrote the paper. Kristien De Paepe ran the PHAR-QA consortium. Constantin Mircioiu played a major role in the statistical analyses of the data. Antonio Sánchez Pozo and Dimitrios Rekkas developed the questionnaire. Antonio Sánchez Pozo, Dimitrios Rekkas, Jouni Hirvonen, Borut Bozic, Annie Marcincal and Agnieska Skowron helped with distribution of the survey. Antonio Sánchez Pozo and Borut Bozic provided useful criticism and suggestions during revision of the manuscript, as did Daisy Volmer, Keith Wilson and Kristien De Paepe. Chris van Schravendijk assured the contacts with MEDINE2.

Conflicts of Interest: The authors declare no conflict of interest.

Appendix A. Ranking of Competences by Industrial and Community Pharmacists. (Seq.: Sequential Numbering (as in Figures).

Cluster	Seq.	Competence	Industrial Pharmacists	Community Pharmacists
Cluster 7. Personal competences: learning and knowledge.			83.6	79.2
	1	Ability to identify learning needs and to learn independently (including continuous professional development (CPD)).	93.3	89.8
	2	Analysis: ability to apply logic to problem solving, evaluating pros and cons and following up on the solution found.	97.0	91.1
	3	Synthesis: capacity to gather and critically appraise relevant knowledge and to summarise the key points.	92.4	87.9
	4	**Capacity to evaluate scientific data in line with current scientific and technological knowledge.**	**88.1**	**75.8**
	5	Ability to interpret preclinical and clinical evidence-based medical science and apply the knowledge to pharmaceutical practice.	71.5	75.9
	6	**Ability to design and conduct research using appropriate methodology.**	**57.6**	**40.2**
	7	Ability to maintain current knowledge of relevant legislation and codes of pharmacy practice.	84.6	91.7
Cluster 8. Personal competences: values.			91.7	93.7
	8	Demonstrate a professional approach to tasks and human relations.	93.9	94.5
	9	Demonstrate the ability to maintain confidentiality.	96.9	95.3
	10	Take full personal responsibility for patient care and other aspects of one's practice.	86.7	94.8
	11	Inspire the confidence of others in one's actions and advice.	86.0	88.8
	12	Demonstrate high ethical standards.	94.7	95.2
Cluster 9. Personal competences: communication and organizational skills.			78.7	76.3
	13	Effective communication skills (both orally and written).	89.3	94.8
	14	Effective use of information technology.	86.3	86.1
	15	Ability to work effectively as part of a team.	89.1	89.2
	16	Ability to identify and implement legal and professional requirements relating to employment (e.g., for pharmacy technicians) and to safety in the workplace.	82.2	81.0
	17	Ability to contribute to the learning and training of staff.	77.1	82.5
	18	**Ability to design and manage the development processes in the production of medicines.**	**72.8**	**43.2**
	19	Ability to identify and manage risk and quality of service issues.	78.9	79.2
	20	Ability to identify the need for new services.	62.9	64.5
	21	Ability to communicate in English and/or locally relevant languages.	85.2	74.1

22	Ability to evaluate issues related to quality of service.	80.2	77.9
23	Ability to negotiate, understand a business environment and develop entrepreneurship.	61.2	64.1
Cluster 10. Personal competences: knowledge of different areas of the science of medicines.		63.8	66.1
24	**Plant and animal biology.**	23.3	**39.3**
25	**Physics.**	33.3	**21.7**
26	General and inorganic chemistry.	53.1	43.9
27	Organic and medicinal/pharmaceutical chemistry.	76.7	66.0
28	**Analytical chemistry.**	67.2	**41.9**
29	General and applied biochemistry (medicinal and clinical).	71.9	68.8
30	**Anatomy and physiology; medical terminology.**	70.3	**88.7**
31	Microbiology.	59.2	72.2
32	Pharmacology including pharmacokinetics.	88.4	94.7
33	**Pharmacotherapy and pharmaco-epidemiology.**	75.8	**94.3**
34	**Pharmaceutical technology including analyses of medicinal products.**	84.4	**62.0**
35	Toxicology.	65.1	74.0
36	**Pharmacognosy.**	37.5	**66.5**
37	Legislation and professional ethics.	86.8	89.5
Cluster 11. Personal competences: understanding of industrial pharmacy.		70.7	59.7
38	**Current knowledge of design, synthesis, isolation, characterization and biological evaluation of active substances.**	57.1	**41.7**
39	**Current knowledge of good manufacturing practice (GMP) and of good laboratory practice (GLP).**	81.9	**59.4**
40	**Current knowledge of European directives on qualified persons (QPs).**	66.7	**43.7**
41	**Current knowledge of drug registration, licensing and marketing.**	84.1	**55.7**
42	Current knowledge of good clinical practice (GCP).	63.5	64.5
Cluster 12. Patient care competences: patient consultation and assessment.		52.0	77.0
43	**Ability to perform and interpret medical laboratory tests.**	44.4	**65.5**
44	**Ability to perform appropriate diagnostic or physiological tests to inform clinical decision making e.g., measurement of blood pressure.**	40.9	**73.6**
45	Ability to recognise when referral to another member of the healthcare team is needed because a potential clinical problem is identified (pharmaceutical, medical, psychological or social).	71.9	91.7

Cluster	#	Competence		
Cluster 13. Patient care competences: need for drug treatment.			66.0	87.0
	46	Retrieval and interpretation of relevant information on the patient's clinical background.	63.3	84.0
	47	Retrieval and interpretation of an accurate and comprehensive drug history if and when required.	69.6	91.5
	48	Identification of non-adherence and implementation of appropriate patient intervention.	63.8	86.8
	49	Ability to advise to physicians and—in some cases—prescribe medication.	66.7	87.6
Cluster 14. Patient care competences: drug interactions.			69	93
	50	Identification, understanding and prioritization of drug-drug interactions at a molecular level (e.g., use of codeine with paracetamol).	70.4	91.6
	51	Identification, understanding, and prioritization of drug-patient interactions, including those that preclude or require the use of a specific drug (e.g., trastuzumab for treatment of breast cancer in women with HER2 overexpression).	64.9	89.7
	52	Identification, understanding, and prioritization of drug-disease interactions (e.g., NSAIDs in heart failure).	71.7	96.6
Cluster 15. Patient care competences: provision of drug product.			73.1	83.3
	53	Familiarity with the bio-pharmaceutical, pharmacodynamic and pharmacokinetic activity of a substance in the body.	70.4	81.2
	54	Supply of appropriate medicines taking into account dose, correct formulation, concentration, administration route and timing.	85.2	94.9
	55	Critical evaluation of the prescription to ensure that it is clinically appropriate and legal.	77.6	94.0
	56	Familiarity with the supply chain of medicines and the ability to ensure timely flow of drug products to the patient.	71.1	84.6
	57	Ability to manufacture medicinal products that are not commercially available.	60.6	60.5
Cluster 16. Patient care competences: patient education.			64.0	85.0
	58	Promotion of public health in collaboration with other actors in the healthcare system.	62.8	82.6
	59	Provision of appropriate lifestyle advice on smoking, obesity, *etc.*	57.1	80.9
	60	Provision of appropriate advice on resistance to antibiotics and similar public health issues.	73.0	93.1

Cluster 17. Patient care competences: provision of information and service.			73.0	93.0
	61	**Ability to use effective consultations to identify the patient's need for information.**	68.5	90.9
	62	**Provision of accurate and appropriate information on prescription medicines.**	80.9	94.4
	63	**Provision of informed support for patients in selection and use of non-prescription medicines for minor ailments (e.g., cough remedies...).**	70.9	94.0
Cluster 18. Patient care competences: monitoring of drug therapy.			74.0	86.0
	64	**Identification and prioritization of problems in the management of medicines in a timely manner and with sufficient efficacy to ensure patient safety.**	76.9	93.0
	65	Ability to monitor and report to all concerned in a timely manner, and in accordance with current regulatory guidelines on Good Pharmacovigilance Practices (GVPs), Adverse Drug Events and Reactions (ADEs and ADRs).	81.1	83.4
	66	**Undertaking of a critical evaluation of prescribed medicines to confirm that current clinical guidelines are appropriately applied.**	65.1	80.6
Cluster 19. Patient care competences: evaluation of outcomes.			54.0	70.0
	67	**Assessment of outcomes on the monitoring of patient care and follow-up interventions.**	60.2	79.0
	68	Evaluation of cost effectiveness of treatment.	47.3	61.2

Notes: Competences in bold are those showing a statistically significant difference in distribution of rankings between groups (chi-square, $p < 0.05$).

References

1. Atkinson, J.; Nicholson, J.; Rombaut, B. Survey of pharmaceutical education in Europe—PHARMINE—Report on the integration of the industry component in pharmacy education and training. *Ind. Pharm.* **2012**, *13*, 17–20.
2. Atkinson, J.; Rombaut, B. The 2011 PHARMINE report on pharmacy and pharmacy education in the European Union. *Pharm. Pract.* **2011**, *9*, 169–187. [CrossRef]
3. The International Pharmaceutical Federation (FIP). Global pharmacy workforce report. 2012. Available online: http://www.fip.org/humanresources (accessed on 5 October 2015).
4. *Ordre des Pharmaciens de France. Pharmaciens de L'industrie des Médicaments et Produits de Santé*, Available online: http://www.ordre.pharmacien.fr/index.php/Communications/Publications-ordinales/Livret-d-accueil-de-la-section-B (accessed on 5 October 2015).
5. The European Union. The Council Directive of 16 September 1985 concerning the coordination of provisions laid down by law, regulation or administrative action in respect of certain activities in the field of pharmacy. Available online: http://eur-lex.europa.eu/legal-content/EN/TXT/PDF/?uri=CELEX:31985L0432&from=EN (accessed on 5 October 2015).
6. The European Union. The EU directive 2013/55/EU on the recognition of professional qualifications. Availabe online: http://eur-lex.europa.eu/LexUriServ/LexUriServ.do?uri=OJ:L:2005:255:0022:0142:EN:PDF (accessed on 5 October 2015).
7. The European Union directive 2001/83/EC of the European parliament and of the council of 6 November 2001 on the community code relating to medicinal products for human use. Available online: http://ec.europa.eu/health/documents/eudralex/index_en.htm (accessed on 5 October 2015).
8. The PHARMINE country profile on Pharmacy Education and Training in Germany. Available online: http://www.pharmine.org/wp-content/uploads/2014/05/PHARMINE-WP7-Survey-Germany.pdf (accessed on 5 October 2015).
9. The PHAR-QA project: Quality assurance in European pharmacy education and training. Available online: http://www.phar-qa.eu (accessed on 5 October 2015).
10. Survey Software, Inc. The Survey System. Available online: http://www.surveysystem.com/sscalc.htm (accessed on 5 October 2015).
11. Atkinson, J.; de Paepe, K.; Sánchez Pozo, A.; Rekkas, D.; Volmer, D.; Hirvonen, J.; Bozic, B.; Skowron, A.; Mircioiu, C.; Marcincal, A.; *et al.* The PHAR-QA Project: Competency framework for pharmacy practice—First steps, the results of the European network Delphi Round 1. *Pharmacy* **2015**, *3*, 307–329. [CrossRef]
12. The Bologna Process. The European Higher Education Area. Available online: http://www.ehea.info/ (accessed on 5 October 2015).
13. Marz, R.; Dekker, F.W.; van Schravendijk, C.; O'Flynn, S.; Ross, M.T. Tuning research competences for Bologna three cycles in medicine: Report of a MEDINE2 European consensus survey. *Perspect. Med. Educ.* **2013**, *2*, 181–195. Available online: http://download-v2.springer.com/static/pdf/799/art%253A10.1007%252Fs40037-013-0066-z.pdf?token2=exp=1429779128~acl=%2Fstatic%2Fpdf%2F799%2Fart%25253A10.1007%25252Fs40037-013-0066-z.pdf*~hmac=8cc61f57990544e852082e9749b6e580c1306f08bbab0d086.4cc9b01433864f8 (accessed on 5 October 2015). [CrossRef] [PubMed]
14. Leik, R.K. A measure of ordinal consensus. *Pac. Soc. Rev.* **1966**, *9*, 85–90. [CrossRef]
15. GraphPad Software, Inc. GraphPad statistical pack. Available online: http://www.graphpad.com/ (accessed on 5 October 2015).
16. Qualitative data systems analysis. Qualitative data analysis software (QSR). Available online: http://www.qsrinternational.com/products_nvivo.aspx (accessed on 5 October 2015).
17. Elvey, R.; Hassel, K.; Hall, J. Who do you think you are? Pharmacists' perceptions of their professional activity. *Int. J. Pharm. Pract.* **2013**, *13*, 322–332. [CrossRef] [PubMed]

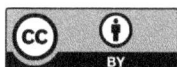

pharmacy

MDPI

Article
How Do European Pharmacy Students Rank Competences for Practice?

Jeffrey Atkinson [1,2,*], Kristien De Paepe [3], Antonio Sánchez Pozo [4], Dimitrios Rekkas [5], Daisy Volmer [6], Jouni Hirvonen [7], Borut Bozic [8], Agnieska Skowron [9], Constantin Mircioiu [10], Annie Marcincal [11], Andries Koster [12], Keith Wilson [13], Chris van Schravendijk [14] and Sandra Hočevar [15]

1   Pharmacology Department, Lorraine University, 5 rue Albert Lebrun, 54000 Nancy, France
2   Pharmacolor Consultants Nancy, 12 rue de Versigny, 54600 Villers, France
3   Pharmacy Faculty, Vrije Universiteit Brussel, Laarbeeklaan 103, Brussels 1090, Belgium; kdepaepe@vub.ac.be
4   Faculty of Pharmacy, University of Granada, Campus Universitario de la Cartuja s/n, Granada 18701, Spain; sanchezpster@ugr.com
5   School of Pharmacy, National and Kapodistrian University Athens, Panepistimiou 30, Athens 10679, Greece; rekkas@pharm.uoa.gr
6   Pharmacy Faculty, University of Tartu, Nooruse 1, Tartu 50411, Estonia; daisy.volmer@ut.ee
7   Pharmacy Faculty, University of Helsinki, Yliopistonkatu 4, P.O. Box 33-4, Helsinki 00014, Finland; jouni.hirvonen@helsinki.fi
8   Faculty of Pharmacy, University of Ljubljana, Askerceva cesta 7, Ljubljana 1000, Slovenia; Borut.Bozic@ffa.uni-lj.si
9   Pharmacy Faculty, Jagiellonian University, Golebia 24, Krakow 31-007, Poland; askowron@cm-uj.krakow.pl
10 Pharmacy Faculty, University of Medicine and Pharmacy "Carol Davila" Bucharest, Dionisie Lupu 37, Bucharest 020021, Romania; constantin.mircioiu@yahoo.com
11 Faculty of Pharmacy, European Association of Faculties of Pharmacy, Université de Lille 2, Lille 59000, France; annie.marcincal@pharma.univ-lille2.fr
12 Department of Pharmaceutical Sciences, European Association of Faculties of Pharmacy, Utrecht University, PO Box 80082, 3508 TB Utrecht, The Netherlands; A.S.Koster@uu.nl
13 School of Life and Health Sciences, Aston University, Birmingham, B47ET, UK; k.a.wilson@aston.ac.uk
14 Medical Faculty, Vrije Universiteit Brussel, Laarbeeklaan 103, 1090 Brussels, Belgium; chrisvs@vub.ac.be
15 European Pharmacy Students' Association (EPSA), Rue de Luxembourg 19/6, 1000 Brussels, Belgium; sandra.hoce@gmail.com
*   Correspondence: jeffrey.atkinson@univ-lorraine.fr; Tel./Fax: +33-383-273-703

Academic Editor: Yvonne Perrie
Received: 14 September 2015; Accepted: 15 January 2016; Published: 26 January 2016

Abstract: European students ($n = 370$), academics ($n = 241$) and community pharmacists ($n = 258$) ranked 13 clusters of 68 personal and patient care competences for pharmacy practice. The results show that ranking profiles for all three groups as a rule were similar. This was especially true of the comparison between students and community pharmacists concerning patient care competences suggesting that students have a good idea of their future profession. A comparison of first and fifth (final) year students shows more awareness of patient care competences in the final year students. Differences do exist, however, between students and community pharmacists. Students—like academics—ranked competences concerned with industrial pharmacy and the quality aspects of preparing drugs, as well as scientific fundamentals of pharmacy practice, well above the rankings of community pharmacists. There were no substantial differences amongst rankings of students from different countries although some countries have more "medicinal" courses than others. This is to our knowledge the first paper to look at how, within a healthcare sectoral profession such as pharmacy, the views on the relative importance of different competences for practice of those educating the future professionals and their students, are compared to the views of working professionals.

Pharmacy **2016**, *4*, 8

Keywords: pharmacy; education; competences; framework; student; practice

1. Introduction

The PHARMINE (Pharmacy education in Europe) [1] study aimed at promoting the use of competence frameworks in European pharmacy education. Competence frameworks have been developed to facilitate practitioner development and assessment, and have already been used in the workplace to monitor and improve practice of Singaporean hospital pharmacists [2], and of hospital pharmacists in Queensland [3]. Studies have also been conducted in the UK [4] and in Canada [5] in community pharmacy. These studies attempted to define the roles of pharmacists in a community or hospital setting and establish measurable outcomes on the possible impact of the application of competence frameworks for development and assessment. All studies concluded that competence frameworks are useful tools to monitor and improve performance in the workplace. PHARMINE and its follow-up project PHAR-QA (Quality Assurance in European Pharmacy Education and Training) [6] extended this approach to pharmacy education. A competence framework similar to that used in the four studies cited previously was used. The main difference between the two was, that with the four studies done in the workplace, the emphasis was on the fourth level of Miller's triangle *i.e.*, *"does"* whereas in this study emphasis was one the first two levels *"knows"* and *"knows how"* (see conclusions). Thus the studies in the workplace are aimed at personal development and improvement in action whereas this study is aimed more at adapting pharmacy education to a competence approach. These aspects will be taken up in the discussion following the exposé of the study and results.

The PHAR-QA ("Quality Assurance in European PHARmacy Education and Training") project, funded by the European Commission, asked pharmacy students, academics, and community pharmacists to rank competences for pharmacy practice.

This paper asks the question of whether the ranking of competences by students is similar to that of academics and/or to that of community pharmacists. It also looks at whether their ideas on the relative ranking of competences evolve during their studies by comparing the scores of first year students with that of fifth (final) year students. Finally, it also looks at potential differences amongst students from different countries.

The methodology used is based on that in the MEDINE ("Medical Education in Europe") project that asked medical doctors and students to rank competences for the medical practitioner [7].

2. Experimental Section

Ranking data on competences for practice were obtained via the PHAR-QA surveymonkey [8] questionnaire that was available online from 14 February 2014 through 1 November 2014 *i.e.*, 8.5 month [9]. Respondents came from 33/38 (Table 1) countries drawn from the European Higher Education Area [10].

Table 1. Student respondents by country.

The number of students who responded from each country.	
Germany	127
Czech Republic	32
Portugal	28
Romania	21
Belgium	20
Finland	18
Macedonia (FYROM)	12

Table 1. *Cont.*

The number of students who responded from each country.	
Croatia	10
Malta	10
France	7
Latvia	7
Montenegro	7
Estonia	6
Greece	6
Poland	6
Slovenia	6
Spain	6
Norway	5
The Netherlands	5
Turkey	5
UK	4
Serbia	3
Switzerland	3
Austria	2
Denmark	2
Sweden	2
Ukraine	2
Albania	1
Bosnia	1
Hungary	1
Kosovo	1
Lithuania	1
Slovakia	1
Belarus	0
Bulgaria	0
Iceland	0
Ireland	0
Italy	0

Nine countries were represented by 10 or more respondents, 21 countries by four or more, five countries had no respondents. Two respondents did not answer the "country of residence" question. The questionnaire was distributed by several means. Firstly the PHAR-QA consortium nominated four regional managers (north, south, east, and west) who sent out the survey to the various countries based on their geographical location in Europe. The regional managers contacted pharmacy departments, students and organizations representing other groups, chambers, governments and other agencies. The survey was also distributed by the European Pharmacy Students' Association via its national representatives. Thus the survey was distributed randomly and anonymously. No attempt was made to target specific groups to obtain a previously established number of respondents, as a function, for example, of the population of the country. Our approach produced an imbalanced distribution across European countries with small countries such as Malta in the top nine for respondents and large countries such as Italy having no student respondents. Furthermore no attempt was made to have an equal number of respondents for the three groups (students, academics, community pharmacists) from a given country. It was felt, however, that what the survey lost in balance it gained in being random and anonymous.

The first six questions of the survey were on the profile of the respondent asking, amongst others, country of residence, current occupation (student, academic, community pharmacist), and, for students, year of study.

Questions 7 through 19 asked about 13 clusters of competences with a total of 68 competences. Questions in clusters 7 through 11 were concerned with personal competences and in clusters 12 through 19 with patient care competences (Table A1).

Respondents were asked to rank the proposals for competences with a 4-point Likert scale (Table 2).

Table 2. Ranking of competences.

Rank	Significance	Explanation
1	Not important	Can be ignored
2	Quite important	Valuable but not obligatory
3	Very important	Obligatory, with exceptions depending upon field of pharmacy practice
4	Essential	Obligatory

There was also a "cannot rank" possibility as well as the possibility of leaving the answer blank; these numbers were pooled.

Results are presented in the form of "scores": score = (frequency rank 3 + frequency rank 4) as % of total frequency. This calculation is based on that used by the MEDINE consortium [11] that studied the ranking of competences for medical practice by academics and medical students. Scores were used for descriptive purposes only.

Leik ordinal consensus, an indication of the ordinal dispersion characterization of the intra-group frequencies [12] was calculated using an in-house excel spreadsheet. Responses for Leik ordinal consensus were graded as they were in the MEDINE study:

- < 0.2 poor,
- $0.21 - 0.4$ fair,
- $0.41 - 0.6$ moderate,
- $0.61 - 0.8$ substantial,
- > 0.81 good.

Data for the three groups were analyzed at three levels: overall, cluster of competences, and individual competences. Data comparing first and fifth year students were analyzed at the competence level. Data comparing scores from five countries with an arbitrarily chosen number of respondents $\geqslant 20$ (see Table 1), with the nature or the content of the pharmacy course was also analyzed at the competence level only. The nature of the course was defined on the basis of the hours spent on medicinal and chemical sciences [13] and given as an index "medicinal/chemical score" = (% of total course hours spent on medicinal subjects /% of total course hours spent on chemical subjects). Medicinal subjects included pharmacology, therapeutics, *etc.*, and chemical subjects included analytical chemistry, organic chemistry, *etc.* The full list of subjects in each is given in the paper on heterogeneity on pharmacy education in Europe cited previously. Data were also compared to the course content: the relative amounts of time spent on lectures and on traineeship (data from the PHARMINE study).

The significance of differences between the results for ranking by groups was established using the chi-square test on the distribution of frequencies for the four ranks. A significance level of $p < 0.05$ was used (chi-square for three degrees of freedom (4 ranks $-$ 1) = 7.81; *ns* = not significant).

Data is presented mainly as star plots. Star plots are suited to display multivariate ordinal observations with an arbitrary number of variables. This representation is suitable for the study of clusters as well as for detecting outliers [14].

All statistical tests were performed using GraphPad software [15].

3. Results and Discussion

The first level of analysis was the overall analysis of the pooled results ($n = 68$ competences). In Table 3 is given the distribution of rankings. For all three groups the response rate was high with only 6.9% to 11.7% unable to reply. This suggests that all groups of respondents considered they were sufficiently informed to reply to the questions asked.

Table 3. Overall distribution (over 68 competences) of rankings by students, community pharmacists, and academics.

	Students		Community Pharmacists		Academics	
Number of respondents	370		258		241	
Theoretical total number of replies	25,160 (= 370 × 68)		17,544 (= 258 × 68)		16,388 (= 241 × 68)	
Replies by rank	Frequency	%	Frequency	%	Frequency	%
4	8428	33.5	6643	37.9	5821	35.5
3	8967	35.6	6002	34.2	6005	36.6
2	4278	17.0	3076	17.5	2982	18.2
1	531	2.1	608	3.5	366	2.2
Cannot rank + blanks	619	11.7	1215	6.9	1214	7.4
Score (%)	77.4		78.3		77.9	
Leik ordinal consensus	0.59		0.55		0.58	

Scores for the three groups were similar and within the range of means of 77.4% to 78.3% showing that almost 80% of the competences proposed were considered "obligatory for practice" by all.

Values for Leik's ordinal consensus were similar (0.55–0.59) and at the top end of the "moderate" grade (0.41–0.6). It should be noted, however, that this particular Leik analysis confounds groups and competences. Thus ordinal consensus may be moderate because there are differences amongst the groups and/or amongst the competences. Albeit as judged from the Leik ordinal consensus values, dispersion was relatively low. This suggests that groups were relatively homogeneous and there were no subgroups with responses significantly different from the others. Similar values for ordinal consensus were reported by the MEDINE consortium when they evaluated the ranking of competences for medical doctors. Their respondent population consisted of two-thirds academics delivering undergraduate medical education, and 28% medical students (see MEDINE citations above).

The second level of analysis was based on the grouping of competences into clusters representing the major domains of practice. In Figure 1 are given the scores for the 13 clusters of competences (numbered 7 through 19).

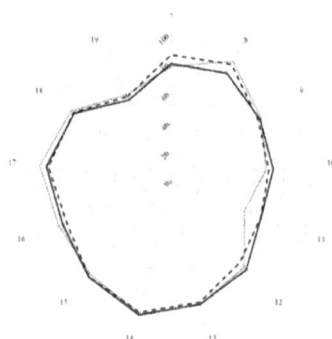

Figure 1. Scores (central vertical axe, 0%–100%) for the 13 (numbered 7 through 19) clusters of competences of students (full line), academics (dashed line), and community pharmacists (dotted line).

Scores for most clusters were 80% or above. Scores were lower than 80% for clusters of personal competences especially those for cluster 11 that dealt with industrial pharmacy. In this case, students had similar scores to academics (chi-square: 2.85, *ns*) and scored well above community pharmacists (chi-square: 89.04, $p < 0.05$). Students scored lower than academics for personal competence clusters 7 and 8, and lower than community pharmacists for cluster 8. Scores were also lower for cluster 19 (evaluation of outcomes) with no difference between students and academics (chi-square: 1.79, *ns*) or community pharmacists (chi-square: 3.19, *ns*).

In Figure 2 are given the values for Leik's ordinal consensus for the 13 clusters of competences (numbered 7 through 19).

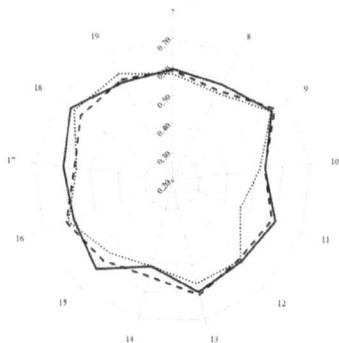

Figure 2. Leik's ordinal consensus (central vertical axe, 0.2–0.7) for the 13 clusters of competences of students (full line), academics (dashed line), and community pharmacists (dotted line).

For most clusters, ordinal consensus was at the top end of the 0.41–0.60 "moderate" category. Students (and academics) generally showed higher values than community pharmacists and this was especially true for cluster 11 which community pharmacists scored low (Figure 1) and showed a low ordinal consensus (Figure 2). This suggests that the low score for cluster 11 was not shared by all community pharmacists.

The third level of analysis was at the level of competences. In Figure 3 are given the scores for the 68 competences (numbered 1 through 68 on the circumference). This figure shows that more detail amongst the groups is revealed by analysis at this third, competence level.

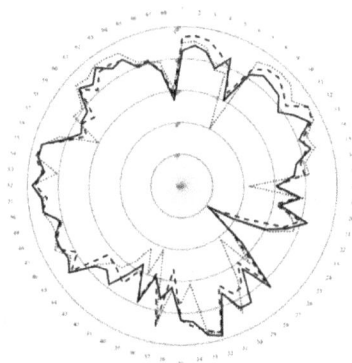

Figure 3. Scores (central vertical axe, 0%–100%) for the 68 competences of students (full line), academics (dashed line), and community pharmacists (dotted line).

Significant differences between students and community pharmacists (Table A1) were seen in cluster 8 "personal competences 8–12: values" covering aspects such as contact, confidentiality, responsibility and ethics for which student scores were lower than those of community pharmacists.

This was also seen but to lesser extent in the comparison between students and academics. Student scores for quality aspects of drug production and testing were higher than those of community pharmacists—cluster 11 (industrial pharmacy, competences 38–42) and competence 57 in cluster 15 "ability to manufacture medicinal products that are not commercially available". It may be worthwhile in the future to consider focus groups in order to ascertain when and why do community pharmacists change their perspective on those competences (38–42) related to industrial pharmacy. Differences between students and academics were seen in cluster 7 "personal competences 1–7: learning and knowledge"; competences 1, 3, and 4 dealing with ability to learn independently and critical appraisal of relevant knowledge were scored lower by students.

Although competence 6 dealing with research issues was scored low by students (and by academics) the score was significantly higher than that of community pharmacists. This lack of recognition that pharmacy is a research-based discipline is paralleled by the lack of a substantial link between biomedical research and medical education and practice as described in the MEDINE study [16]. In the latter paper, Van Schravendijk and his MEDINE colleagues suggested ways of strengthening this link by bibliographic research and thesis work during pre-graduate study.

Such tools do exist in many pharmacy departments. In some cases this "science" aspect is taken even further with traineeships based on participation in clinical research topics in community and hospital pharmacy, and in pharmaceutical research and development in industrial settings. Further efforts are needed to promote such activities at a wider postgraduate level. Emphasis on such aspects in continuing professional development could help maintain the research-based nature of pharmacy.

Globally, the ranking by students, academics, and community pharmacists were similar. Patient care competences were ranked similarly by students and community pharmacists suggesting, importantly, that students have a good conception of their future job responsibilities and practice. Because there were few differences between academics and community pharmacists, it is also important to notice that academics have a good conception of the activity in community pharmacy. This critical nature of the "type of patient care provided by pharmacists" has been emphasized following evaluation of competences for pharmacists on a world-wide basis [17].

In Figure 4 are given the values for Leik's ordinal consensus for the 13 clusters of competences (numbered 7 through 19).

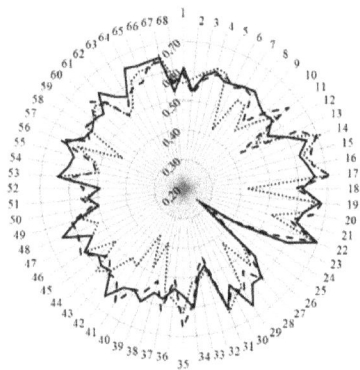

Figure 4. Leik's ordinal consensus (central vertical axe, 0.2–0.7) for the 68 competences of students (full line), academics (dashed line), and community pharmacists (dotted line).

For many competences ordinal consensus was lower in community pharmacists than in both students and academics. Ordinal consensus was low for all groups for "competences" 24 "biology" and 25 "physics". These are, however, "subjects" not "competences".

Figure 5 shows the ranking scores for first ($n = 30$) and fifth ($n = 77$) students. Competences 24, 25, 26, 35, 36, 38, and 43 decreased in ranking from the first to the fifth year, whereas 4, 22, 31, 37, 39, 59, 63, and 65 increased.

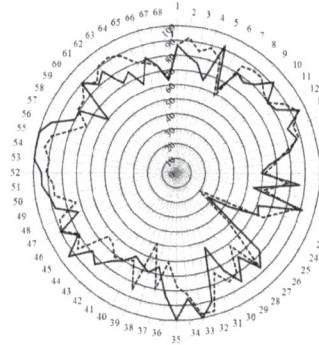

Figure 5. Ranking scores (central vertical axe, 0%–100%) for the 68 competences (on the circumference) by first (full line) and fifth (dotted line) year students.

The evolution of ranking throughout the pharmacy degree course, reflected by the changes in ranking between first and fifth year students, involved mainly personal values and subject areas. Ranks were fifth year > first year for competences 4, 22, 31, 37, and 39, and first year > fifth year for competences 24, 25, 26, 35, 36, 38, and 43. Three patient care competences increased in ranking throughout studies and these were 59 "provision of appropriate lifestyle advice on smoking, obesity, *etc.*", 63 "provision of informed support for patients in selection and use of non-prescription medicines for minor ailments (e.g., cough remedies)", and 65 "ability to monitor and report to all concerned in a timely manner, and in accordance with current regulatory guidelines on Good Pharmacovigilance Practices (GVPs), Adverse Drug Events and Reactions (ADEs and ADRs)". This may be linked to the increased awareness of advanced students of their role as an advisor on health matters, especially so once they have undergone their traineeship in their final year.

One final aspect concerns possible differences in results overall between participants from different countries. In Figure 6 are given the rankings for five countries in which the respondent number was ≥ 20.

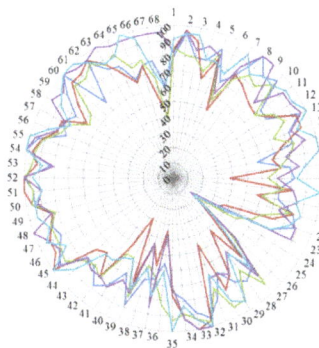

Figure 6. Rankings for five countries in which the respondent number was ≥ 20. Belgium: dark blue; Czech Republic: red; Germany: green; Portugal: mauve; Romania: light blue.

Although the overall patterns of the rankings showed no large discrepancies amongst the different countries, there were significant differences in the mean scores (Table 4) with the Czech Republic giving the lowest score (73%) and Romania the highest (84%).

Table 4. Mean scores for five countries shown in Figure 6 together with data for course nature (= time spent on traineeship/time spent on lectures) and course content (= time spent on medicinal subjects/time spent on chemical subjects). Data from Atkinson (2014) and PHARMINE (2014) cited previously.

Country	Mean Ranking Score (%, $n = 68$ Competences)	Course Nature	Course Content
		Time Spent on Traineeship/Time Spent on Lectures	Time Spent on Medicinal Subjects/Time Spent on Chemical Subjects
Belgium	80	0.75	1.13
Czech Republic	73	0.76	1.12
Germany	78	1.25	0.71
Portugal	83	0.84	1.64
Romania	84	0.66	0.95

Although there are substantial differences in course nature and content this was not reflected in mean scores (Table 3) or in the patterns of the rankings (Figure 6). Some differences were observed: for example, students of the Czech Republic gave low scores for competence 18 (ability to design and manage the development processes in the production of medicines) and competence 40 (current knowledge of European directives on qualified persons (QPs)), but this was not observed for Belgium which has a similar course nature and content.

4. Conclusions

To our knowledge, this is the first study in which students in a sectoral profession are asked to rank the relative importance of competences for practice in their future professional lives. Globally, their perception of the relative importance of competences is similar to that of practicing community pharmacists especially in the area of patient care competences.

Given the growing interest in competence-based educational reforms in several areas of the world, it would be useful to do studies similar to this one in various areas worldwide in order to see whether student perceptions are equally advanced in all areas. This could be done through European-funded programs such as Erasmus+ [18] and would be one way of increasing awareness of and developing competence-based education in other regions. The results of such studies could be linked to the education framework used to train future pharmacists in those countries.

A proviso to this study is that it concentrates on community pharmacy practice. Whilst 70%–80% of pharmacists work in a community pharmacy in Europe (data from PHARMINE), many work in other areas such as hospital and industrial pharmacy. As education for jobs in the latter areas differs substantially amongst European countries, and the options for hospital and industrial pharmacy courses and training occur late in the courses it proved impossible to do a study similar to this in the specific areas of hospital or industrial pharmacy.

Another proviso is that, given the diversity of country of origin, it would have been useful to know something about the level of English proficiency for cohorts from different counties as the survey was delivered in English and if proficiency in English had any impact on the results. It would have been interesting to have information on the English proficiency, via for example, scores in the "Test of English as a Foreign Language (TOEFL)" examination [19]. However this is not uniformly applied in Europe and not even uniformly applied within each member state. We can comment that students ranked competence 21 "ability to communicate in English" very highly (score 85) suggesting that they at least recognized the necessity to understand English. It should be noted that the consortium strived to make the questions understandable to non-native English speakers.

Furthermore, when asked to rank subject areas listed in the European Directive many were ranked as "not important/can be ignored". These are not competences [20] as such but components of competences (see Miller's triangle, below). They were included in the questionnaire because they are cited in the European directive on the sectoral profession of pharmacy [21].

The final question to be discussed relates to how a competence framework could be incorporated into pharmacy education. This will be discussed in relation to Miller's triangle that describes a conceptual, pyramidal model of the various facets of competence, in his case applied to clinical practice [22] (Figure 7).

The studies cited in the introduction on the use of competency frameworks for the improvement of performance are mostly concerned with the fourth level of this triangle—"does/action" whereas in this paper we are equally concerned with the other three levels, especially the first two "knows and knows how". Given the low scores of most of the subject areas included in cluster 10, it would appear that students (as well as academics and community pharmacist practitioners) do not fully grasp the importance of some subjects as building blocks of the competences required for practice. This also outlines the fact that the simple inclusion of subject areas within a European regulatory directive is not a fully sufficient way to ensure the teaching and acquirement of competences for practice. One of the functions or uses of the PHAR-QA framework could be therefore to provide a road-book for the development of integrated, coordinated courses that groups several subject areas under a broad competence heading. The way in which this is to be carried out need not be harmonized or imposed by European directives or other legislative means but could be left to the wisdom of individual faculties to find solutions. Another function of the PHAR-QA competence framework could be as a basis of accreditation at level 2 of the Miller's triangle allowing a more realistic evaluation of a student based on his/her competence to synthesise the different subject areas into a comprehensive understanding of different competences. This entails a switch in evaluation from normative procedures that rank candidates with arbitrary cut-off points to competence-referenced testing that evaluates whether a candidate is (or is not) ready to pass onto a higher level. The way in which this is developed would again be up to individual faculties. It should be noted that changing the method of evaluation is often a good beginning for a change in courses.

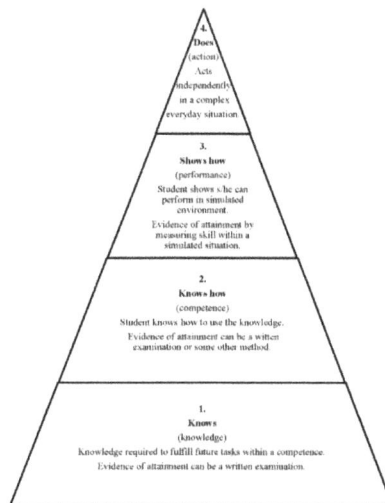

Figure 7. Miller's triangle.

The PHAR-QA framework could also be used at the third level in the performance testing of students. Here one could also use the patient substitutes (or "standardized" patients as described by Miller cited previously). Such "patients" would present students with elements such as symptoms, prescriptions, *etc.* calling upon their competences to solve problems related to drug interactions, for example. How this would be constructed and run would again by up to the individual faculty. It should also be noticed that a change to a competency-based assessment would logically abandon a fixed time traineeship ship at level 3, as is specified by the EU directive and adopted by all EU countries at the present time, and its replacement by a system whereby the student would remain at level 3 in traineeship until s/he has shown to be competent enough to pass to level 1 and exercise his/her profession [23]. Whilst not going to such an extreme, it can be acknowledged that there is a (sometimes large) gap between levels 1 through 3 and level 4 or between the more theoretical academic approach and the real-life work situation. This could be addressed in junior pharmacists using the PHAR-QA framework as a basis for work-based self-directed learning and case-based assignments set and monitored by a senior colleague (see the Rutter, *et al.* reference cited in the introduction).

Acknowledgments: With the support of the Lifelong Learning program of the European Union: 527194-LLP-1-2012-1-BE-ERASMUS-EMCR. This project has been funded with support from the European Commission. This publication reflects the views only of the author; the Commission cannot be held responsible for any use which may be made of the information contained therein.

Author Contributions: Jeffrey Atkinson constructed, ran and analyzed the survey and wrote the paper. Kristien De Paepe ran the PHAR-QA consortium. Constantin Mircioiu played a major role in the statistical analyses of the data. Antonio Sanchez-Pozo and Dimitri Rekkas developed the questionnaire. Antonio Sanchez-Pozo, Dimitri Rekkas, Jouni Hirvonen, Borut Bozic, Annie Marcincal, and Agneska Skowron helped with distribution of the survey. Antonio Sanchez-Pozo, Daisy Volmer, and Kristien De Paepe provided useful criticism and suggestions during revision of the manuscript. Chris van Schravendijk assured the contacts with MEDINE. Sandra Hočevar played a major role in distributing the survey to students.

Conflicts of Interest: The authors declare no conflicts of interest.

Appendix

Table A1. Ranking scores for competences by groups (students, academics, community pharmacists). Note that the numbering of the clusters of competences starts at 7, *i.e.*, after the 6 questions on profile of respondent. N: number of competence. Stud.: students. Acad.: academics. Comm.: community pharmacists. Chi: chi-square. *vs.*: *versus*.

	N	Competence	Stud.	Acad.	Chi Stud. *vs.* Acad.	Comm.	Chi Stud. *vs.* Comm.
	1	Ability to identify learning needs and to learn independently (including continuous professional development (CPD)).	84.5	93.7	15.7	89.8	13.1
	2	Analysis: ability to apply logic to problem solving, evaluating pros and cons and following up on the solution found.	88.8	94.5	7.5	91.1	3.6
Cluster 7. Personal competences: learning and knowledge.	3	Synthesis: capacity to gather and critically appraise relevant knowledge and to summarise the key points.	85.1	92.8	10.8	87.9	4.0
	4	Capacity to evaluate scientific data in line with current scientific and technological knowledge.	76.5	87.3	18.5	75.8	0.4
	5	Ability to interpret preclinical and clinical evidence-based medical science and apply the knowledge to pharmaceutical practice.	86.0	81.2	5.2	75.9	17.3
	6	Ability to design and conduct research using appropriate methodology.	60.6	65.4	4.9	40.2	34.3

Table A1. *Cont.*

	N	Competence	Stud.	Acad.	Chi Stud. *vs.* Acad.	Comm.	Chi Stud. *vs.* Comm.
	7	Ability to maintain current knowledge of relevant legislation and codes of pharmacy practice.	81.7	86.3	3.3	91.7	25.7
	8	Demonstrate a professional approach to tasks and human relations.	86.6	91.5	7.7	94.5	23.3
	9	Demonstrate the ability to maintain confidentiality.	85.4	92.3	22.8	95.3	50.6
Cluster 8. Personal competences: values.	10	Take full personal responsibility for patient care and other aspects of one's practice.	84.4	88.3	3.2	94.8	24.9
	11	Inspire the confidence of others in one's actions and advice.	77.8	83.8	8.9	88.8	13.0
	12	Demonstrate high ethical standards.	85.3	95.3	43.4	95.2	24.6
	13	Effective communication skills (both orally and written).	91.2	93.5	3.9	94.8	4.0
	14	Effective use of information technology.	81.1	83.8	1.4	86.1	3.8
	15	Ability to work effectively as part of a tea.	86.4	83.3	6.1	89.2	1.1
	16	Ability to identify and implement legal and professional requirements relating to employment (e.g., for pharmacy technicians) and to safety in the workplace.	74.8	77.9	1.9	81.0	4.5
Cluster 9. Personal competences: communication and organisational skills.	17	Ability to contribute to the learning and training of staff.	73.5	79.6	6.6	82.5	6.6
	18	Ability to design and manage the development processes in the production of medicines.	61.2	60.0	0.8	43.2	38.0
	19	Ability to identify and manage risk and quality of service issues.	77.5	76.1	4.0	79.2	2.3
	20	Ability to identify the need for new services.	65.0	61.8	7.7	64.5	1.2
	21	Ability to communicate in English and/or locally relevant languages.	84.5	79.6	2.3	74.1	16.3
	22	Ability to evaluate issues related to quality of service.	73.0	71.0	3.5	77.9	7.4
	23	Ability to negotiate, understand a business environment and develop entrepreneurship.	62.2	46.4	15.6	64.1	2.0
	24	Plant and animal biology.	38.8	31.1	5.1	39.3	1.0
	25	Physics.	20.9	25.6	2.3	21.7	0.8
	26	General and inorganic chemistry	53.0	45.6	3.3	43.9	5.3
	27	Organic and medicinal/pharmaceutical chemistry.	86.3	80.2	10.8	66.0	37.0
	28	Analytical chemistry	65.8	60.0	3.0	41.9	46.9
Cluster 10. Personal competences: knowledge of different areas of the science of medicines.	29	General and applied biochemistry (medicinal and clinical).	85.4	74.2	10.8	68.8	22.6
	30	Anatomy and physiology; medical terminology.	85.2	75.8	11.2	88.7	3.3
	31	Microbiology.	72.2	67.0	3.3	72.2	1.5
	32	Pharmacology including pharmacokinetics.	97.5	95.6	3.7	94.7	3.0
	33	Pharmacotherapy and pharmaco-epidemiology.	95.3	92.5	3.1	94.3	2.2
	34	Pharmaceutical technology including analyses of medicinal products.	86.9	89.0	1.4	62.0	50.8
	35	Toxicology.	85.0	84.4	17.3	74.0	27.7
	36	Pharmacognosy.	65.9	52.9	11.3	66.5	2.1
	37	Legislation and professional ethics.	71.7	88.8	26.8	89.5	44.2

Table A1. *Cont.*

	N	Competence	Stud.	Acad.	Chi Stud. *vs.* Acad.	Comm.	Chi Stud. *vs.* Comm.
Cluster 11. Personal competences: understanding of industrial pharmacy.	38	Current knowledge of design, synthesis, isolation, characterisation and biological evaluation of active substances.	59.9	57.5	1.9	41.7	34.2
	39	Current knowledge of good manufacturing practice (GMP) and of good laboratory practice (GLP).	79.2	75.4	1.6	59.4	29.8
	40	Current knowledge of European directives on qualified persons (QPs).	55.3	59.2	1.8	43.7	39.9
	41	Current knowledge of drug registration, licensing and marketing.	65.7	72.1	4.6	55.7	11.9
	42	Current knowledge of good clinical practice (GCP).	78.1	68.2	9.1	64.5	23.8
Cluster 12. Patient care competences: patient consultation and assessment.	43	Ability to perform and interpret medical laboratory tests.	72.0	65.3	5.9	65.5	6.0
	44	Ability to perform appropriate diagnostic or physiological tests to inform clinical decision making e.g., measurement of blood pressure.	76.1	64.5	17.3	73.6	7.8
	45	Ability to recognise when referral to another member of the healthcare team is needed because a potential clinical problem is identified (pharmaceutical, medical, psychological or social).	91.7	89.1	2.2	91.7	9.5
Cluster 13. Patient care competences: need for drug treatment.	46	Retrieval and interpretation of relevant information on the patient's clinical background.	85.6	79.3	8.4	84.0	0.7
	47	Retrieval and interpretation of an accurate and comprehensive drug history if and when required.	87.6	89.4	5.1	91.5	2.3
	48	Identification of non-adherence and implementation of appropriate patient intervention.	87.1	85.8	6.1	86.8	24.5
	49	Ability to advise to physicians and—in some cases—prescribe medication.	81.9	80.7	2.5	87.6	5.3
Cluster 14. Patient care competences: drug interactions.	50	Identification, understanding and prioritisation of drug-drug interactions at a molecular level (e.g., use of codeine with paracetamol).	91.4	91.8	1.1	91.6	0.6
	51	Identification, understanding, and prioritisation of drug-patient interactions, including those that preclude or require the use of a specific drug (e.g., trastuzumab for treatment of breast cancer in women with HER2 overexpression).	91.4	87.7	4.4	89.7	5.0
	52	Identification, understanding, and prioritisation of drug-disease interactions (e.g., NSAIDs in heart failure).	97.0	94.5	8.9	96.6	2.7

Table A1. *Cont.*

	N	Competence	Stud.	Acad.	Chi Stud. *vs.* Acad.	Comm.	Chi Stud. *vs.* Comm.
Cluster 15. Patient care competences: provision of drug product.	53	Familiarity with the bio-pharmaceutical, pharmacodynamic and pharmacokinetic activity of a substance in the body.	89.3	90.8	3.5	81.2	11.6
	54	Supply of appropriate medicines taking into account dose, correct formulation, concentration, administration route and timing.	94.3	96.3	16.3	94.9	18.0
	55	Critical evaluation of the prescription to ensure that it is clinically appropriate and legal.	93.9	94.1	6.6	94.0	11.1
	56	Familiarity with the supply chain of medicines and the ability to ensure timely flow of drug products to the patient.	81.6	78.6	4.5	84.6	11.3
	57	Ability to manufacture medicinal products that are not commercially available.	74.1	69.0	1.5	60.5	21.2
Cluster 16. Patient care competences: patient education.	58	Promotion of public health in collaboration with other actors in the healthcare system.	75.8	75.1	1.1	82.6	5.9
	59	Provision of appropriate lifestyle advice on smoking, obesity, *etc.*	76.9	71.0	3.8	80.9	4.7
	60	Provision of appropriate advice on resistance to antibiotics and similar public health issues.	90.3	89.4	5.2	93.1	3.6
Cluster 17. Patient care competences: provision of information and service.	61	Ability to use effective consultations to identify the patient's need for information.	85.6	81.1	3.1	90.9	11.1
	62	Provision of accurate and appropriate information on prescription medicines.	92.7	89.3	8.0	94.4	11.0
	63	Provision of informed support for patients in selection and use of non-prescription medicines for minor ailments (e.g., cough remedies).	85.7	89.4	1.7	94.0	14.4
Cluster 18. Patient care competences: monitoring of drug therapy.	64	Identification and prioritisation of problems in the management of medicines in a timely manner and with sufficient efficacy to ensure patient safety.	88.5	87.9	8.2	93.0	8.7
	65	Ability to monitor and report to all concerned in a timely manner, and in accordance with current regulatory guidelines on Good Pharmacovigilance Practices (GVPs), Adverse Drug Events and Reactions (ADEs and ADRs).	79.8	80.9	5.0	83.4	3.3
	66	Undertaking of a critical evaluation of prescribed medicines to confirm that current clinical guidelines are appropriately applied.	80.7	81.6	0.3	80.6	4.5
Cluster 19. Patient care competences: evaluation of outcomes.	67	Assessment of outcomes on the monitoring of patient care and follow-up interventions.	73.3	73.7	0.5	79.0	4.4
	68	Evaluation of cost effectiveness of treatment.	53.3	57.7	2.1	61.2	4.8

Chi-square, d. f. 3, p = 0.05: 7.8. The chi-square test was performed on the frequencies of rankings.

References

1. The PHARMINE (*Pharmacy Education in Europe*) consortium. Work programme 3: Final Report Identifying and Defining Competences for Pharmacists. Available online: http://www.pharmine.org/wp-content/uploads/2014/05/PHARMINE-WP3-Final-ReportDEF_LO.pdf (accessed on 12 January 2016).
2. Rutter, V.; Wong, C.; Coombes, I.; Cardiff, L.; Duggan, C.; Yee, M.L.; Lim, K.W.; Bates, I. Use of a General Level Framework to Facilitate Performance Improvement in Hospital Pharmacists in Singapore. *Am. J. Pharm. Educ.* **2012**, *76*, 1–10. Available online: http://www.ajpe.org/action/doSearch?AllField=bates (accessed on 12 January 2016). [CrossRef] [PubMed]

3. Coombes, I.; Avent, M.; Cardiff, L.; Bettenay, K.; Coombes, J.; Whitfield, K.; Stokes, J.; Davies, G.; Bates, I. Improvement in Pharmacist's Performance Facilitated by an Adapted Competency-Based General Level Framework. *J. Pharm. Pract. Res.* **2010**, *40*, 111–118. Available online: http://onlinelibrary.wiley.com/doi/10.1002/j.2055–2335.2010.tb00517.x/abstract (accessed on 12 January 2016). [CrossRef]

4. Antoniou, S.; Webb, D.G.; Mcrobbie, D.; Davies, J.G.; Bates, I.P. A controlled study of the general level framework: Results of the South of England competency study. *Pharm. Educ.* **2005**, *5*, 1–8. Available online: http://pharmacyeducation.fip.org/pharmacyeducation/article/view/171/146 (accessed on 12 January 2016). [CrossRef]

5. Winslade, N.E.; Tamblyn, R.M.; Taylor, L.K.; Schuwirth, L.W.T.; Van der Vleuten, C.P.M. Integrating Performance Assessment, Maintenance of Competence, and Continuing Professional Development of Community Pharmacists. *Am. J. Pharm. Educ.*; 2007; 71, pp. 1–9. Available online: http://www.ncbi.nlm.nih.gov/pmc/journals/383/ (accessed on 12 January 2016). [CrossRef]

6. The PHAR-QA Project. Quality Assurance in European Pharmacy Education and Training. Available online: www.phar-qa.eu (accessed on 12 January 2016).

7. Medical Education in Europe. Available online: http://medine2.com/ (accessed on 12 January 2016).

8. The Survey Software—The Survey System. Available online: http://www.surveysystem.com/sscalc.htm (accessed on 12 January 2016).

9. Atkinson, J.; de Paepe, K.; Sánchez Pozo, A.; Rekkas, D.; Volmer, D.; Hirvonen, J.; Bozic, B.; Skowron, A.; Mircioiu, C.; Marcincal, A.; *et al.* The PHAR-QA Project: Competency Framework for Pharmacy Practice—First Steps, the Results of the European Network Delphi Round 1. *Pharmacy* **2015**, *3*, 307–329. Available online: http://www.mdpi.com/2226-4787/3/4/307 (accessed on 12 January 2016). [CrossRef]

10. The European Higher Education Area. Available online: http://www.ehea.info/ (accessed on 12 January 2016).

11. Marz, R.; Dekker, F.W.; Van Schravendijk, C.; O'Flynn, S.; Ross, M.T. Tuning research competences for Bologna three cycles in medicine: Report of a MEDINE2 European Consensus Survey. *Perp. Med. Educ.*; 2013; 2, pp. 181–195. Available online: http://www.ncbi.nlm.nih.gov/pmc/articles/PMC3792236/ (accessed on 12 January 2016). [CrossRef] [PubMed]

12. Leik, R.K. A measure of ordinal consensus. *Pac. Soc. Rev.* **1966**, *9*, 85–90. Available online: http://www.jstor.org/stable/1388242 (accessed on 12 January 2016). [CrossRef]

13. Atkinson, J. Heterogeneity of Pharmacy Education in Europe. *Pharmacy* **2014**, *2*, 231–243. Available online: http://www.mdpi.com/search?q=&journal=pharmacy&volume=&page=&authors=atkinson&section=&issue=&number=&article_type=&special_issue=&search=Search (accessed on 12 January 2016). [CrossRef]

14. Chambers, J.; Cleveland, W.; Kleiner, B.; Tukey, P. Graphical Methods for Data Analysis. *J. Appl. Stat.* **1984**, *11*, 233–234. Available online: http://www.tandfonline.com/doi/abs/10.1080/02664768400000024?journalCode=cjas20#.VciiCocbCpo (accessed on 12 January 2016).

15. The GraphPad Statistical Pack. Available online: http://www.graphpad.com/ (accessed on 12 January 2016).

16. Van Schravendijk, C.; Marz, R.; Garcia-Sloane, J. Exploring the integration of the biomedical research component in undergraduate medical education. *Med. Teach.* **2013**, *35*, e1243–e1251. Available online: http://informahealthcare.com/doi/pdfplus/10.3109/0142159X.2013.768337 (accessed on 12 January 2016). [CrossRef] [PubMed]

17. Bruno, A.; Bates, I.; Brock, T.; Anderson, C. Towards a Global Competency Framework. *Am. J. Pharm. Educ.*; 2010; 74, pp. 1–2. Available online: http://www.ncbi.nlm.nih.gov/pmc/articles/PMC2865424/ (accessed on 12 January 2016). [CrossRef]

18. The Erasmus+. EU Programme for Education, Training, Youth and Sport. Available online: http://ec.europa.eu/programmes/erasmus-plus/index_en.htm (accessed on 12 January 2016).

19. TOEFL—Test of English as a Foreign Language. Available online: http://www.ets.org/toefl (accessed on 12 January 2016).

20. Fernandez, N.; Dory, V.; Ste-Marie, L.G.; Chaput, M.; Charlin, B.; Boucher, A. Varying conceptions of competence: An Analysis of how Health Sciences Educators Define Competence. *Med. Educ.* **2012**, *46*, 357–365. Available online: http://onlinelibrary.wiley.com/doi/10.1111/j.1365–2923.2011.04183.x/abstract (accessed on 12 January 2016). [CrossRef] [PubMed]

21. The EU Directive 2013/55/EU on the Recognition of Professional Qualifications. Available online: http://eur-lex.europa.eu/LexUriServ/LexUriServ.do?uri=OJ:L:2005:255:0022:0142:EN:PDF (accessed on 12 January 2016).

22. Miller, G.E. The assessment of clinical skills/competences/performance. *Acad. Med.* **1990**, *65*, 63–67. Available online: http://winbev.pbworks.com/f/Assessment.pdf (accessed on 26 January 2016). [CrossRef]

23. Carr, S.J. Assessing clinical competency in medical senior house officers: How and Why Should We Do it? *Postgrad. Med. J.* **2004**, *80*, 63–66. Available online: http://pmj.bmj.com/content/80/940/63.full.pdf+html. (accessed on 12 January 2016). [CrossRef] [PubMed]

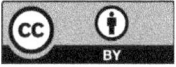

pharmacy

MDPI

Article

Does the Subject Content of the Pharmacy Degree Course Influence the Community Pharmacist's Views on Competencies for Practice?

Jeffrey Atkinson [1,2,*], Kristien De Paepe [3], Antonio Sánchez Pozo [4], Dimitrios Rekkas [5], Daisy Volmer [6], Jouni Hirvonen [7], Borut Bozic [8], Agnieska Skowron [9], Constantin Mircioiu [10], Annie Marcincal [11], Andries Koster [12], Keith Wilson [13], Chris van Schravendijk [14] and Jamie Wilkinson [15]

[1] Pharmacology Department, Lorraine University, 5 rue Albert Lebrun, 54000 Nancy, France
[2] Pharmacolor Consultants Nancy, 12 rue de Versigny, Villers 54600, France
[3] Department of Pharmacy, Vrije Universiteit Brussel, Laarbeeklaan 103, Brussels 1090, Belgium; kdepaepe@vub.ac.be
[4] Faculty of Pharmacy, University of Granada (UGR), Campus Universitario de la Cartuja s/n, Granada 18701, Spain; sanchezp@ugr.es
[5] School of Pharmacy, National and Kapodistrian University Athens, Panepistimiou 30, Athens 10679, Greece; rekkas@pharm.uoa.gr
[6] Pharmacy Faculty, University of Tartu, Nooruse 1, Tartu 50411, Estonia; daisy.volmer@ut.ee
[7] Pharmacy Faculty, University of Helsinki, Yliopistonkatu 4, P.O. Box 33-4, Helsinki 00014, Finland; jouni.hirvonen@helsinki.fi
[8] Faculty of Pharmacy, University of Ljubljana, Askerceva cesta 7, Ljubljana 1000, Slovenia; Borut.Bozic@ffa.uni-lj.si
[9] Pharmacy Faculty, Jagiellonian University, UL, Golebia 24, Krakow 31-007, Poland; askowron@cm-uj.krakow.pl
[10] Pharmacy Faculty, University of Medicine and Pharmacy "Carol Davila" Bucharest, Dionisie Lupu 37, Bucharest 020021, Romania; constantin.mircioiu@yahoo.com
[11] European Association of Faculties of Pharmacy, Faculty of Pharmacy, Université de Lille 2, Lille 59000, France; annie.marcincal@pharma.univ-lille2.fr
[12] European Association of Faculties of Pharmacy, Department Pharmaceutical Sciences, Utrecht University, PO Box 80082, 3508 TB Utrecht, The Netherlands; A.S.Koster@uu.nl
[13] School of Life and Health Sciences, Aston University, Birmingham, B4 7ET, UK; k.a.wilson@aston.ac.uk
[14] Vrije Universiteit Brussel, Laarbeeklaan 103, 1090 Brussels, Belgium; chrisvs@vub.ac.be
[15] Pharmaceutical Group of the European Union (PGEU), Rue du Luxembourg 19, 1000 Brussels, Belgium; j.wilkinson@pgeu.eu
*   Author to whom correspondence should be addressed; jeffrey.atkinson@univ-lorraine.fr; Tel./Fax: +33-383-27-37-03.

Academic Editor: Reem Kayyali
Received: 16 July 2015; Accepted: 17 August 2015; Published: 1 September 2015

Abstract: Do community pharmacists coming from different educational backgrounds rank the importance of competences for practice differently—or is the way in which they see their profession more influenced by practice than university education? A survey was carried out on 68 competences for pharmacy practice in seven countries with different pharmacy education systems in terms of the relative importance of the subject areas chemical and medicinal sciences. Community pharmacists were asked to rank the competences in terms of relative importance for practice; competences were divided into personal and patient-care competences. The ranking was very similar in the seven countries suggesting that evaluation of competences for practice is based more on professional experience than on prior university education. There were some differences for instance in research-related competences and these may be influenced, by education.

Keywords: pharmacy; education; community; practice; competence

Pharmacy **2015**, *3*, 137–153

1. Introduction

In 1985, the then European Economic Community (EEC) published a directive [1] on pharmacy practice that assumed that pharmacy education in the EEC was broadly comparable and, thus, that the European education system was producing pharmacists with similar competences. In the early 1990s, the European Association of Faculties of Pharmacy (EAFP) [2] questioned these assumptions [3]. EAFP surveyed pharmacy courses in the 11 EEC members and found that although the emphasis in most faculties was on chemical sciences, there was great variability in pharmacy degree courses in the EEC regarding the percentages of time spent on different subjects [4].

At that time it was hoped that European integration would produce greater harmonization in pharmacy education and therefore in competences for practice. In 2011, the PHARMINE (*"PHARMacy Education IN Europe"*) project [5] revisited this problem. In the 20-year interval between the two studies there was a shift in several countries from chemical to medicinal sciences, albeit, overall variability in degree courses from country to country had not decreased [6]. PHARMINE reflected upon whether differences in pharmacy degrees could be minored by expressing content as competences rather than subjects.

As a follow-up to PHARMINE, a second study, the PHAR-QA (*"Quality Assurance in European PHARmacy-Education and Training"*) project [7], again funded by the European Commission, asked community pharmacists to rank competences for pharmacy practice.

This paper combines the results of the PHARMINE and PHAR-QA studies. It looks at whether the nature of the degree course (in terms of the relative importance of the subject areas chemical and medicinal sciences taken as an indication of a more "scientific" or a more "clinical" course) has any influence on the way in which community pharmacists ranked the competences they consider are required for practice. The paper evaluates to what extent university education or professional experience can influence the way in which practicing community pharmacists judge their *métier* and how the balance between these two factors could be altered by the introduction of competence-based education.

2. Experimental Section

In the PHARMINE project, country profiles for pharmacy education and training were drawn up with the help of academics, students, professional pharmacists, and their organizations, as well as representatives of different governmental bodies concerned with pharmacy in the 47 countries of the European Higher Education Area [8]. Amongst others, one of the areas explored in the country profiles was the structure of the pharmacy degree course that was divided into six subject areas: chemical sciences, medicinal sciences, biological sciences, pharmaceutical technology, and law and societal issues. A subject area course index was calculated as: ((percentage of contact hours spent on medicinal subjects/percentage of contact hours spent on chemical subjects) x 100) using data from the PHARMINE study, as given in the 2014 paper on heterogeneity of pharmacy education cited above [6].

In the PHARMINE study, "medicinal subjects" included contact hours in the subjects of anatomy, physiology, medical terminology, pathology, histology, nutrition, pharmacology/pharmacotherapy, toxicology, hematology, immunology, parasitology, hygiene, emergency therapy, non-pharmacological treatment, clinical chemistry/bio-analysis, radiochemistry, dispensing process, drug prescription, prescription analysis (detection of adverse effects and drug interactions), generic drugs, planning, running and interpretation of the data, of clinical trials, medical devices, orthopedics, over the counter medicines, complementary therapy, at-home support and care, skin illness and treatment, homeopathy, phyto-therapy, drugs in veterinary medicine, pharmaceutical care, pharmaceutical therapy of illness, and disease. "Chemical subjects" included contact hours in the subjects of general and inorganic chemistry, medical physico-chemistry, organic chemistry, pharmacopeia analysis, analytical chemistry, and pharmaceutical chemistry including analysis of medicinal products.

Ranking data on competences for practice were taken from the PHAR-QA *surveymonkey* [9] questionnaire that was available online from 14 January 2014 to 1 November 2014 *i.e.*, 8.5 months. Contacts were made by electronic and other means with the same groups as in the PHARMINE study (see previously). *Post hoc* analysis of the data allowed the creation of six subgroups: academics, students, community pharmacists, hospital pharmacists, industrial pharmacists, and pharmacists working in other areas. Here we will present the data for community pharmacists; data for other professional categories will be presented elsewhere [10].

The first six questions of the PHAR-QA survey were on the profile of the respondent asking, amongst others, country of residence, current occupation, and duration of activity.

Questions seven through 19 asked about 13 groups of competences with a total of 68 competences (see annex). Questions in groups seven through 11 were concerned with personal competences and in groups 12 through 19 with patient care competences.

Respondents were asked to rank the proposals for competences with a Likert scale:

1. Not important = Can be ignored.
2. Quite important = Valuable but not obligatory.
3. Very important = Obligatory with exceptions depending upon field of pharmacy practice.
4. Essential = Obligatory.

Results are presented in the form of "scores" based on the methodology used in MEDINE2 [11]: score = (frequency rank 3 + frequency rank 4) as % of total frequency. Scores give more granularity and a better pictorial representation than the basic Likert data. Data were obtained from 39 European countries. Data presented here are from the seven European Union member states in which the number of respondents was > 10 (Table 1). Analysis was limited to the European Union as its 28 member states come under the directive on sectoral professions such as pharmacy [12]. One of the annexes of this directive lists the subject areas that are to be taught in the pharmacy degree course in the European Union. Of the 28 member states only seven provided 10 or more community pharmacists respondents.

Statistical Analysis

Results are also expressed as medians with 25 and 75% percentiles; differences among countries were analyzed using the Kruskal-Wallis test followed by Dunn's multiple comparisons test. All statistics were performed using GraphPad software [13].

3. Results and Discussion

In Table 1 are the medians for duration of practice. Kruskal-Wallace analysis showed a significant effect of country ($P = 0.0014$) and the Dunn's multiple comparisons test showed that the duration of practice of the respondents from the Czech Republic was lower than that of respondents from Germany, Ireland or Spain. None of the other comparisons were significant.

Table 1 also shows the medicinal sciences/chemical sciences scores. In Germany the degree course is more "chemical"; in Belgium, the Czech Republic, and Spain the importance of the two subject areas is equal; in The Netherlands and the United Kingdom there is a more "medicinal" course, and this is even more pronounced in Ireland. The medicinal/chemical ratio varies almost four-fold from Germany (0.7) to Ireland (2.6).

Finally, Table 1 shows overall the median rankings for competences ($n = 68$). The Kruskal-Wallis test showed a significant difference amongst countries ($P = 0.0006$) with a significantly higher median for Spain compared to Belgium, Germany, and Ireland. None of the other multiple comparisons amongst countries reached statistical significance.

Table 1. Characteristics of the seven countries, the medicinal sciences/chemical sciences indices (latter data from the PHARMINE study), and the rankings for competences.

Country	Number of respondents	Duration of activity (years; median, 25% and 75% percentiles)	Medicinal sciences %	Chemical sciences %	Medicinal/chemical score	Ranking of competences (median, 25% and 75% percentiles, $n = 68$)
Belgium	25	10/5/20	24	27	1.1	81/63/91
Czech Republic	15	5/5/15	19	17	1.1	84/67/92
Germany	13	30/15/30	28	40	0.7	82/67/92
Ireland	13	20/10/33	36	14	2.6	77/55/92
Spain	27	15/10/30	28	24	1.2	91/82/96
The Netherlands	18	20/5/23	31	20	1.6	82/57/94
United Kingdom	48	10/5/20	24	14	1.7	87/59/96

Figure 1 shows the ranking by the seven countries of the 68 competences. This is presented as a radar chart. Radar charts are a useful way to display multivariate observations with an arbitrary number of variables. It allows one to find clusters and also to identify outliers [14]. This radar chart presentation allows an easy overview of the global rankings of competences. It underlines the fact that overall the global rankings by the different countries are similar, with similar highs and lows. This is especially true for the left-hand side of the Figure that represents the rankings for the patient care competences (number 43 through 68). Opinions of the relative importance of such competences appear to be formed by work experience rather than university education. In answer to the question "do community pharmacists coming from different educational backgrounds rank the importance of competences for practice differently" the answer would be no in the case of patient care competences. Examination of Figure 1 shows that the ranking of competences for practice is very similar in seven countries that have different systems of pharmacy education. It should be noted that the ranking score is based on a combination of ranks 3 and 4 that specify that competences are "obligatory".

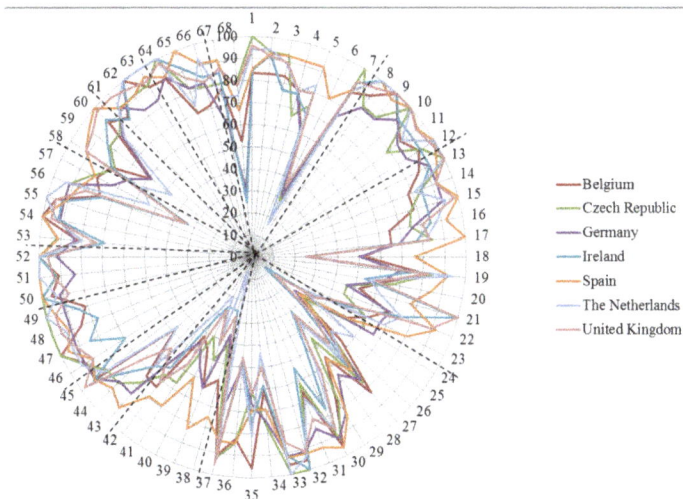

Figure 1. Radar chart of the ranking scores (on the central vertical axe, 0%–100%) for the 68 competences (on the circumference) by the seven countries (in different colours). Dotted lines separate the 13 competence groups (see annex) in Figure 1 are given the ranking scores for the 68 competences by the seven countries.

There are more differences in the right-hand side of the Figure that represents personal competences. Competence 6 is an interesting case. The difference between minimum and maximum for country rankings in group 7 ("personal competences: learning and knowledge") competence 6 ("ability to design and conduct research using appropriate methodology") was large (63, see Table A1); Spain, which has a "balanced" course with a medicinal sciences/chemical sciences index of 1.2, ranked highest with 80%. Ireland and the Netherlands which have more "medical" indices of 2.6 and 1.6, respectively, showed the lowest rankings for competence 6: 18 and 17%, respectively. Spain also ranked highest for all competences. In the research-related group 11 ("personal competences: understanding of industrial pharmacy") Spain scored highest for all 5 competences. Thus differences for Spain may be influenced by education rather than professional experience, albeit, Germany, which has a more "chemical" index (0.7), did not rank competence 6 or the competences in group 11 particularly high.

Several provisos should be added. It is possible that differences in ranking scores are related to duration of practice (*i.e.*, numbers of years since leaving university) rather than to course content. With the median years of practice being significantly different it could very well be that older pharmacists in a given country took a very different course of study 30–40 years ago than younger pharmacists from the same country. Furthermore, it is likely the mix of medicinal/chemical subjects would have differed within countries for participants dependent on when they studied especially as there has been a move towards more medicinal sciences in the past 20 years (see introduction). This cannot be tested, however, as numbers in the different groups do not allow the creation of subgroups based on duration of practice. Some comments can be made on the basis of the existing data. The community pharmacist respondents from the Czech Republic were younger than in several other countries, but the Czech Republic community pharmacists did not show any marked differences with other countries as far as ranking of competences was concerned. Spanish community pharmacists did show a specific pattern of ranking in several groups of competences but their median duration of practice was mid-range.

The conclusion of this paper relies on the fact that the curricula investigated are as different as possible in the relative importance of "medicinal" versus "chemical" sciences component. The seven countries selected were selected on the basis of providing more than 10 respondents. Nonetheless they do represent a significantly wide range of scores. Ireland has the highest value of the 26 European Union member states that have pharmacy departments (1st/26), and Germany the 3rd from the lowest (23rd/26)[vi].

The PHARMINE study cited above showed that a competence approach is rarely used in pre-graduate pharmacy education in Europe. There have been several studies on the use of a competence framework to monitor and improve pharmacy practice in a working environment. A study using the general level framework with Singaporean hospital pharmacists showed that all but eight of the 63 behavioral descriptors improved in nine months [15]. A similar study with hospital pharmacists in Queensland showed an improvement in 35 out of 61 competences [16]. Studies have also been conducted in Canada [17]. and elsewhere. The results of all these studies are that competence frameworks are useful tools to monitor and improve performance.

4. Conclusions

This study shows that community pharmacists largely form their opinions on the importance of competences of the basis of work experience rather than university education. The move to harmonize European pharmacy practice expressed in the 1980s seems to have been successful, as judged from the similar way in which community pharmacists from different countries rank competences for practice. However this is less the result of harmonization of pharmacy education that still shows wide diversity.

The short-term perspective of this work is the modification of the existing questionnaire according to the results obtained and the endorsement of the modified version.

The long-term perspective is the introduction of competence-based learning into the university curriculum for pharmacy. This is being discussed in Australia and New Zealand [18] and elsewhere. It now needs to be considered in Europe. Our results suggest that differences in university pharmacy programs are not crucial in the development of specific competencies (at least in the field of community pharmacy, where the majority of pharmacists work). Thus, we do not need a very stringent and tight framework for curricula of pharmacy education. Academia provides graduates with competencies as

Pharmacy **2015**, *3*, 137–153

"novices" (according to five-stage model of competencies proposed by Dreyfus and Dreyfus, 1980 [19]). Thus, competence-based learning in universities would provide a sound foundation allowing graduates to gather experience through practical training in the real job environment. Furthermore, academic freedom as to course content should be incorporated into quality assurance of pharmacy education especially when EU directive is "translated" into national frameworks.

Acknowledgments: With the support of the Lifelong Learning programme of the European Union: 527194-LLP-1-2012-1-BE-ERASMUS-EMCR. This project has been funded with support from the European Commission. This publication reflects the views only of the author; the Commission cannot be held responsible for any use which may be made of the information contained therein.

Author Contributions: Jeffrey Atkinson designed, constructed, ran and analysed the survey and wrote the paper. Kristien De Paepe ran the PHAR-QA consortium. Constantin Mircioiu played a major role in the statistical analyses of the data. Antonio Sánchez Pozo and Dimitrios Rekkas developed the questionnaire. Antonio Sánchez Pozo, Dimitrios Rekkas, Jouni Hirvonen, Borut Bozic, Annie Marcincal and Agnieska Skowron helped with distribution of the survey. Antonio Sánchez Pozo, Daisy Volmer and Kristien De Paepe provided useful criticism and suggestions during revision of the manuscript. Chris van Schravendijk assured the contacts with MEDINE. Jamie Wilkinson played a major role in distributing the survey to community pharmacists.

Conflicts of Interest: The authors declare no conflict of interest.

Appendix A

Table A1. Ranking of competences by countries.

Seq.	Competence	Belgium	Czech Republic	Germany	Ireland	Spain	The Netherlands	United Kingdom	Min.	Max.	Range: max-min.
	Group 7. Personal competences: learning and knowledge										
1	1. Ability to identify learning needs and to learn independently (including continuous professional development (CPD)).	83	100	85	85	85	94	96	83	100	17
2	2. Analysis: ability to apply logic to problem solving, evaluating pros and cons and following up on the solution found.	83	93	92	92	93	94	92	83	94	11
3	3. Synthesis: capacity to gather and critically appraise relevant knowledge and to summarise the key points.	83	93	77	77	93	89	90	77	93	16
4	4. Capacity to evaluate scientific data in line with current scientific and technological knowledge.	78	67	77	77	92	78	79	67	92	25
5	5. Ability to interpret preclinical and clinical evidence-based medical science and apply the knowledge to pharmaceutical practice.	63	73	62	69	92	83	79	62	92	31
6	6. Ability to design and conduct research using appropriate methodology.	33	29	31	18	80	17	36	17	80	63
7	7. Ability to maintain current knowledge of relevant legislation and codes of pharmacy practice.	88	100	75	92	89	89	93	75	100	25
	Group 8. Personal competences: values										
8	1. Demonstrate a professional approach to tasks and human relations.	92	86	85	100	100	100	96	85	100	15
9	2. Demonstrate the ability to maintain confidentiality.	100	86	85	100	96	100	100	85	100	15
10	3. Take full personal responsibility for patient care and other aspects of one's practice.	92	100	92	92	100	100	100	92	100	8
11	4. Inspire the confidence of others in one's actions and advice.	87	79	85	92	96	88	96	79	96	18
12	5. Demonstrate high ethical standards.	92	93	85	92	100	100	98	85	100	15
	Group 9. Personal competences: communication and organisational skills.										
13	1. Effective communication skills (both orally and written).	87	100	92	92	96	100	100	87	100	13

Table A1. *Cont.*

Seq.	Competence	Belgium	Czech Republic	Germany	Ireland	Spain	The Netherlands	United Kingdom	Min.	Max.	Range: max–min.
14	2. Effective use of information technology.	78	85	92	85	92	81	92	78	92	14
15	3. Ability to work effectively as part of a team.	78	77	92	85	100	94	98	77	100	23
16	4. Ability to identify and implement legal and professional requirements relating to employment (e.g., for pharmacy technicians) and to safety in the workplace.	65	75	77	85	92	88	81	65	92	27
17	5. Ability to contribute to the learning and training of staff.	65	85	69	77	100	81	83	65	100	35
18	6. Ability to design and manage the development processes in the production of medicines.	52	25	50	25	76	25	26	25	76	51
19	7. Ability to identify and manage risk and quality of service issues.	82	85	69	75	92	94	83	69	94	25
20	8. Ability to identify the need for new services.	62	67	62	54	85	56	59	54	85	31
21	9. Ability to communicate in English and/or locally relevant languages.	52	46	46	100	77	63	100	46	100	54
22	10. Ability to evaluate issues related to quality of service.	68	46	69	75	92	75	90	46	92	46
23	11. Ability to negotiate, understand a business environment and develop entrepreneurship.	61	58	67	50	81	69	43	43	81	37
	Group 10. Personal competences: knowledge of different areas of the science of medicines.										
24	1. Plant and animal biology.	52	62	67	31	54	27	35	27	67	40
25	2. Physics.	26	31	25	8	27	60	13	8	60	52
26	3. General and inorganic chemistry.	57	46	42	31	46	50	39	31	57	26
27	4. Organic and medicinal/pharmaceutical chemistry.	83	77	75	69	69	63	53	53	83	29
28	5. Analytical chemistry.	57	46	67	31	58	38	33	31	67	36
29	6. General and applied biochemistry (medicinal and clinical).	74	77	83	46	85	56	62	46	85	38
30	7. Anatomy and physiology; medical terminology.	96	92	92	77	96	88	88	77	96	19
31	8. Microbiology.	65	62	83	54	92	69	78	54	92	38
32	9. Pharmacology including pharmacokinetics.	96	100	92	100	92	94	91	91	100	9
33	10. Pharmacotherapy and pharmaco-epidemiology.	96	100	92	92	92	100	85	85	100	15
34	11. Pharmaceutical technology including analyses of medicinal products.	61	77	75	58	69	44	50	44	77	33
35	12. Toxicology.	96	62	67	75	69	81	62	62	96	34

Table A1. *Cont.*

Seq.	Competence	Belgium	Czech Republic	Germany	Ireland	Spain	The Netherlands	United Kingdom	Min.	Max.	Range: max–min.
36	13. Pharmacognosy.	83	85	50	46	85	50	46	46	85	39
37	14. Legislation and professional ethics.	91	92	67	92	85	88	96	67	96	29
	Group 11. Personal competences: understanding of industrial pharmacy.										
38	1. Current knowledge of design, synthesis, isolation, characterisation and biological evaluation of active substances.	58	42	36	25	75	7	28	7	75	68
39	2. Current knowledge of good manufacturing practice (GMP) and of good laboratory practice (GLP).	63	50	64	25	83	43	42	25	83	58
40	3. Current knowledge of European directives on qualified persons (QPs).	47	40	55	25	61	20	27	20	61	41
41	4. Current knowledge of drug registration, licensing and marketing.	42	67	45	33	79	27	57	27	79	53
42	5. Current knowledge of good clinical practice (GCP).	74	67	55	63	79	40	71	40	79	39
	Group 12. Patient care competences: patient consultation and assessment.										
43	1. Ability to perform and interpret medical laboratory tests.	73	77	83	67	92	67	56	56	92	36
44	2. Ability to perform appropriate diagnostic or physiological tests to inform clinical decision making e.g., measurement of blood pressure.	48	85	83	77	88	47	69	47	88	41
45	3. Ability to recognise when referral to another member of the healthcare team is needed because a potential clinical problem is identified (pharmaceutical, medical, psychological or social).	91	85	92	92	92	87	98	85	98	13
	Group 13. Patient care competences: need for drug treatment.										
46	1. Retrieval and interpretation of relevant information on the patient's clinical background.	91	92	92	69	88	93	87	69	93	24
47	2. Retrieval and interpretation of an accurate and comprehensive drug history if and when required.	100	100	92	85	96	93	91	85	100	15
48	3. Identification of non-adherence and implementation of appropriate patient intervention.	86	100	91	77	92	93	96	77	100	23
49	4. Ability to advise to physicians and—in some cases—prescribe medication.	81	100	91	85	96	100	96	81	100	19
	Group 14. Patient care competences: drug interactions.										

Table A1. *Cont.*

Seq.	Competence	Belgium	Czech Republic	Germany	Ireland	Spain	The Netherlands	United Kingdom	Min.	Max.	Range: max–min.
50	1. Identification, understanding and prioritisation of drug-drug interactions at a molecular level (e.g., use of codeine with paracetamol).	95	100	92	100	100	93	87	87	100	13
51	2. Identification, understanding, and prioritisation of drug-patient interactions, including those that preclude or require the use of a specific drug (e.g., trastuzumab for treatment of breast cancer in women with HER2 overexpression).	91	92	83	92	100	100	93	83	100	17
52	3. Identification, understanding, and prioritisation of drug-disease interactions (e.g., NSAIDs in heart failure).	100	100	92	100	100	100	96	92	100	8
	Group 15. Patient care competences: provision of drug product.										
53	1. Familiarity with the bio-pharmaceutical, pharmacodynamic and pharmacokinetic activity of a substance in the body.	82	92	83	69	91	80	73	69	92	22
54	2. Supply of appropriate medicines taking into account dose, correct formulation, concentration, administration route and timing.	100	100	92	92	100	93	96	92	100	8
55	3. Critical evaluation of the prescription to ensure that it is clinically appropriate and legal.	95	92	92	92	91	100	96	91	100	9
56	4. Familiarity with the supply chain of medicines and the ability to ensure timely flow of drug products to the patient.	76	92	92	75	87	93	83	75	93	18
57	5. Ability to manufacture medicinal products that are not commercially available.	81	83	73	33	82	53	34	33	83	50
	Group 16. Patient care competences: patient education.										
58	1. Promotion of public health in collaboration with other actors in the healthcare system.	77	75	67	77	91	60	91	60	91	31
59	2. Provision of appropriate lifestyle advice on smoking, obesity, etc.	59	83	58	85	96	47	93	47	96	49
60	3. Provision of appropriate advice on resistance to antibiotics and similar public health issues.	90	83	82	92	100	80	98	80	100	20
	Group 17. Patient care competences: provision of information and service.										

Seq.: sequential numbering (as in Figure 1); Min.: minimum; Max.: maximum; Note that the numbering of the groups of competences starts at 7, *i.e.*, after the 6 questions on profile.

Table A1. *Cont.*

Seq.	Competence	Belgium	Czech Republic	Germany	Ireland	Spain	The Netherlands	United Kingdom	Min.	Max.	Range: max–min.
61	1. Ability to use effective consultations to identify the patient's need for information.	86	92	92	85	91	93	98	85	98	13
62	2. Provision of accurate and appropriate information on prescription medicines.	100	92	83	100	91	100	95	83	100	17
63	3. Provision of informed support for patients in selection and use of non-prescription medicines for minor ailments (e.g., cough remedies...)	90	92	83	100	96	100	93	83	100	17
	Group 18. Patient care competences: monitoring of drug therapy.										
64	1. Identification and prioritisation of problems in the management of medicines in a timely manner and with sufficient efficacy to ensure patient safety.	90	100	91	100	91	100	98	90	100	10
65	2. Ability to monitor and report to all concerned in a timely manner, and in accordance with current regulatory guidelines on Good Pharmacovigilance Practices (GVPs), Adverse Drug Events and Reactions (ADEs and ADRs).	70	82	82	92	100	73	87	70	100	30
66	3. Undertaking of a critical evaluation of prescribed medicines to confirm that current clinical guidelines are appropriately applied.	71	80	82	85	91	93	82	71	93	22
	Group 19. Patient care competences: evaluation of outcomes.										
67	1. Assessment of outcomes on the monitoring of patient care and follow-up interventions.	78	80	60	85	90	73	87	60	90	30
68	2. Evaluation of cost effectiveness of treatment.	53	80	30	25	67	73	78	25	80	55

Seq.: sequential numbering (as in Figure 1); Min.: minimum; Max.: maximum; Note that the numbering of the groups of competences starts at 7, *i.e.*, after the 6 questions on profile.

References

1. The European Union. The Council Directive of 16 September 1985 concerning the coordination of provisions laid down by law, regulation or administrative action in respect of certain activities in the field of pharmacy. Available online: http://eur-lex.europa.eu/legal-content/EN/TXT/PDF/?uri=CELEX:31985L0432&from=EN (accessed on 28 August 2015).

2. European Association of Faculties of Pharmacy (EAFP). Available online: http://www.eafponline.eu/ (accessed on 28 August 2015).

3. The European Union. ERASMUS Subject Evaluations: Summary Reports of the Evaluation Conferences by Subject Area. Volume 1 pharmacy. Available online: http://eafponline.eu/wp-content/uploads/2013/04/EAFP-report-prepared-In-European-Commission.-Erasmus-Subject-Evaluations-1995.pdf (accessed on 28 August 2015).

4. BERLIN Humboldt University. 2nd European meetings of the faculties, schools and institutes of pharmacy. 27 September 1994. Available online: http://www.pharmine.org/wp-content/uploads/2014/05/2nd-EU-meeting-of-the-faculties-of-pharmacy-Berlin-1994.pdf (accessed on 28 August 2015).

5. Pharmine: pharmacy education in Europe. Available online: http://www.pharmine.org/ (accessed on 28 August 2015).

6. Atkinson, J. Heterogeneity of pharmacy education in Europe. *Pharmacy* **2014**, *2*, 231–243. Available online: http://www.mdpi.com/2226-4787/2/3/231 (accessed on 28 August 2015). [CrossRef]

7. PHAR-QA. The PHAR-QA project: Quality Assurance in European Pharmacy Education and Training. Available online: www.phar-qa.eu (accessed on 28 August 2015).

8. Bologna Process-European Higher Education Area. History. Available online: http://www.ehea.info/article-details.aspx?ArticleId=3 (accessed on 28 August 2015).

9. Surveymonkey survey creation system. Available online: https://www.surveymonkey.com/ (accessed on 28 August 2015).

10. Atkinson, J.; De Paepe, K.; Sánchez Pozo, A.; Rekkas, D.; Volmer, D.; Hirvonen, J.; Bozic, B.; Skowron, A.; Mircioiu, C.; Marcincal, A.; Koster, A.; Wilson, K.; van Schravendijk, C. The PHAR-QA project: Quality Assurance in European Pharmacy Education and Training. *Results of the Eur. Netw. Delphi.* **2015**, in press.

11. Marz, R.; Dekker, F.W.; Van Schravendijk, C.; O'Flynn, S.; Ross, M.T. Tuning research competences for Bologna three cycles in medicine: Report of a MEDINE2 European consensus survey. *Perp. Med. Educ.* **2013**. Available online: http://www.ncbi.nlm.nih.gov/pmc/articles/PMC3792236/ (accessed on 28 August 2015).

12. European University Association (EUA). EUA Briefing Note on Directive 2013/55/EU, containing the amendments to Directive 2005/36/EC on the Recognition of Professional Qualifications. Available online: http://www.eua.be/Libraries/Higher_Education/EUA_briefing_note_on_amended_Directive_January_2014.sflb.ashx (accessed on 28 August 2015).

13. GraphPad statistical pack. Available online: http://www.graphpad.com/ (accessed on 28 August 2015).

14. Chambers, J.; Cleveland, W.; Kleiner, B.; Tukey, P. Graphical Methods for Data Analysis. *J. Appl. Stat.* **1984**, *11*, 233–234. Available online: http://www.tandfonline.com/doi/abs/10.1080/02664768400000024?journalCode=cjas20#.VciiCocbCpo (accessed on 28 August 2015).

15. Rutter, V.; Wong, C.; Coombes, I.; Cardiff, L.; Duggan, C.; Yee, M.-L.; Lim, K.W.; Bates, I. Use of a General Level Framework to Facilitate Performance Improvement in Hospital Pharmacists in Singapore. *Am. J. Pharm. Educ.* **2012**, *76*, 1–10. Available online: http://www.ajpe.org/action/doSearch?AllField=bates (accessed on 28 August 2015). [CrossRef] [PubMed]

16. Coombes, I.; Avent, M.; Cardiff, L.; Bettenay, K.; Coombes, J.; Whitfield, K.; Stokes, J.; Davies, G.; Bates, I. Improvement in Pharmacist's Performance Facilitated by an Adapted Competency-Based General Level Framework. *J. Pharm. Pract. Res.* **2010**, *40*, 111–118. Available online: http://onlinelibrary.wiley.com/doi/10.1002/j.2055-2335.2010.tb00517.x/abstract (accessed on 28 August 2015).

17. Winslade, N.E.; Tamblyn, R.M.; Taylor, L.K.; Schuwirth, L.W.T.; Van der Vleuten, C.P.M. Integrating Performance Assessment, Maintenance of Competence, and Continuing Professional Development of Community Pharmacists. *Am. J. Pharm. Educ.* **2007**, *71*, 1–9. [CrossRef]

18. Stupans, I.; McAllister, S.; Clifford, R.; Hughes, J.; Krasse, I.; March, G.; Owen, S.; Woulf, J. Nationwide collaborative development of learning outcomes and exemplar standards for Australian pharmacy programmes. *Int. J. Pharm. Pract.* **2014**, *24*, 1–9. [CrossRef] [PubMed]
19. Dreyfus, S.E.; Dreyfus, H.L. *A Five-Stage Model of the Mental Activities Involved in Directed Skill Acquisition*; Storming Media: Washington, USA, 1980.

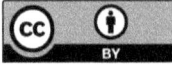

MDPI

St. Alban-Anlage 66

4052 Basel, Switzerland

Tel. +41 61 683 77 34

Fax +41 61 302 89 18

http://www.mdpi.com

MDPI Books Editorial Office

E-mail: books@mdpi.com

http://www.mdpi.com/journal/books

www.ingramcontent.com/pod-product-compliance
Lightning Source LLC
Chambersburg PA
CBHW051905210326
41597CB00033B/6027